S L

The Ultimate Secret
To
Ageless Achievement

Shelia —

May you always
sleep well —

Paul O'Connor

9/20/04

S L E E P

The Ultimate Secret
To
Ageless Achievement

Sufficient, restful sleep is an incredibly important component of any beauty, health or anti-aging regimen. Without it, all products, procedures and programs fall short of their potential.

By
Fawn O'Connor
Anti-Aging Coach

Ronnoco Publishing
PO Box 403, Placentia, CA 92871

This publication is not intended as a diagnosis and/or treatment for any specific sleep disorder. It is intended to provide educational information, ideas and possible solutions for general insomnia. If you are experiencing severe, chronic sleep problems, and/or symptoms of any sleep disorder, by all means seek medical counseling and treatment from a professional health care provider. It is also meant to enlighten our readers as to the many benefits of finding and implementing ways to get sufficient, refreshing sleep.

Sleep – The Ultimate Secret to Ageless Achievement
Copyright © 2002 by Fawn O'Connor

Edited by Mickey Schlatter
Cover Design by Kathi Dunn
Back Cover Writing by Susan Kendrick
Page and Text Design by Laura Rice
Cartoons by Ted Goff
Proofread by Chirayu Borooah and Mickey Schlatter

Printed in the United States by Guardian Printers

Ronnoco Publishing
PO Box 403, Placentia, CA 92831

ISBN 0-9725341-0-5

Dedication

This book is dedicated to my beloved Bill, who started encouraging me to write in 1976, and continued to do so until the time of his sudden death on November 16, 1997. In fact, he actually continued to encourage me after his passing. Almost a year to the day of his transition, I found a letter in his closet that he had written to me after his first heart attack. In the letter, he pleaded with me to follow my dreams, to pursue my goals, and to share with others what I have learned about anti-aging, and self-improvement.

His confidence in me far exceeded my own. It is because of his unwavering belief, that I have had the courage to take the steps I've taken since his transition to the spirit world.

He was the "wind beneath my wings", and still is today.

William J. O'Connor
November 26, 1924 – November 16, 1997

Contents

"Friends are angels who lift us to our feet when our wings have trouble remembering how to fly."

Author Unknown -

Dear Friends,

This is a small book, but it required a large amount of faith, energy and effort to get it written and published. It also required a great deal of advice, support and love from my family, friends, mentors and special angels.

I sincerely hope that the advice and ideas presented here will be of great benefit to you. Being sleep-deprived for many years, and accepting it as inevitable, puts me in the position of realistic empathy for my readers.

My goal . . . my dharma . . . my purpose . . . is to help as many people as possible to look better, feel better and do better. I hope this book will be educational, and motivate you to find a way to get more sleep.

May God bless you with peaceful sleep, productive days and a prosperous consciousness.

Lovingly -

Acknowledgments

"Feeling gratitude and not expressing it is like wrapping a present and not giving it."

William Arthur Ward
American Author/
1921 – 1994

If I expressed the true amount of my gratitude to loved ones, friends and mentors who have been unwavering in their support through this sometimes lonely and laborious, but rewarding, project, this section would be almost as long as the book. Not only have they been supportive with words of encouragement, and an open ear, but incredibly generous with their time, suggestions and feedback.

I will try to be as succinct as it is possible for me to be.

Special Acknowledgment

Dee Hillmer, my precious sister. Your constant expressions of unconditional love, patient listening, and countless phone calls have been more important to my survival than food and water. Thank you for your efforts in helping me make the endless decisions on this book. You're my best friend, and I love you very much.

Norm Hillmer, my dear brother-in-law. You've have always been like a rock, and willing to give me guidance and advice, when asked. Thank you for this, and for not giving it to me when I did not ask, even though I know most of my decisions are out of your comfort zone. Thank you for your love and support.

Lisa Hillmer, my sweet niece, who is always ready, willing and able to eject me from of my computer messes. Thank you for your love and all your help.

Chester Casanave, my very special brother-in-law who has made his transition into the spirit world. He was a prince of a man, and constantly told me,

"You're a very strong woman," at a time when I felt very weak. He continued to reassure me that I could accomplish much more than I thought I could. Guess what, he was right!

My Magnificent Mentors

Webster's Unabridged Dictionary defines a mentor as **"a wise and trusted counselor or teacher."** I have many.

Dr. Frank Richelieu, one of my first mentors. Your incredibly insightful "Living Ideas" programs and audio tapes awakened my spirit to newness at a time when it was totally dead. I've listened to you so many times, that even in the silence of the night, I can hear you saying, **"Don't be afraid to let go of the old, and embrace the new. This is the only way you can bring newness and growth into your life."** Thank you for teaching me this, and a myriad of other priceless lessons.

Deepak Chopra, another early mentor. You have taught me many things, but one of the most important is the wisdom of uncertainty, and to realize that the unknown is just another term for "creation". This lesson has helped me to move into uncharted waters with less anxiety. Also, in "The Seven Spiritual Laws of Success", you enlightened me as to the necessity of finding my daharma, and moving into it without fear or hesitation. You may be pleased to know, I am now in my "daharma."

Bob Schlatter, my writing instructor. His passing into the spirit world is a great loss to all of us who knew him. It is also a great loss to future students who will be denied the opportunity to drink from his cup of knowledge and compassion. Bob was the epitome of what a teacher should be, and convinced me, as a student, that I could definitely write a book.

Dottie Walters, the "grande dame" of the speaking and writing industry. You have been an inspiration from the day I met you. Your incredible knowledge, generosity and courage inspire and motivate me each time I am with you. Thank you for your title suggestion, and for taking the time to read the first draft of this book. Your advice and guidance has been invaluable. You are indeed a true friend, and a consummate mentor.

Mark Victor Hansen, is my "nucleus mentor," and has one of the best marketing minds on the planet. You have been more instrumental in my personal growth and becoming an author than you realize. Thank you for all your incredible seminars, books and cassettes, that have been instruments of my growth. Also thank you for introducing me to mentors like Dottie Walters, Bob Proctor, Dan Poynter, Jack Canfield, Cynthia Kersey, and many more. You see why I refer to you as my "nucleus mentor."

Bob Proctor, one of my most revered mentors. "The Science of Getting Rich" Seminar, sparked a flame in my soul, which was fanned into a raging forest fire by "The Goal Achiever." I am so grateful to have found you at this juncture of my life. Your "insights" into living life to our fullest potential in appreciation for our gifts from our Creator are profound. Thank you for this valuable lesson, and for enlightening me on the process of *expanding my awareness!*

Dan Poynter, the self-publishing guru of the book industry. Thank you for convincing me of the importance of writing this book, and for all of the valuable knowledge you have shared so generously. Your generosity is superceded only by your intelligence. I have learned from your seminars, as well as, from your incredible newsletters. They're awesome!

Brian Tracy, my time management mentor. Thank you for teaching me the value of time management, and how to incorporate this into my life. Also thank you for giving me the permission to share some of what I have learned from you with the readers of this book.

Jim Rohn, mentor to many of my mentors. Thank you for your perception of "Exceptional Living," and for teaching me the importance of self-improvement. Your statement, "Work hard on your job, and you'll earn a living. Work hard on yourself, and you'll earn a fortune."... got my attention!

Jack Canfield, you are indeed the Dean of Self-Esteem. Learning the real reason behind why I did not finish projects was a most valuable lesson. Now that you've enlightened me as to the culprit behind my procrastination, I'm getting things finished. As you can see, I actually did finish this book! Thank you.

Cynthia Kersey, the epitome of a woman who has passion for her work. You are indeed "**Unstoppable,**" and you've convinced me I can be too. Thank you for being such an inspiration.

Other mentors to whom I am grateful are **Zig Zigler, Anthony Robbins and Wayne Dyer,** who are some of the great ones.

Note: Many of my mentors publish informative, motivational and inspirational newsletters, absolutely FREE. Just subscribe. Their web site addresses are listed in the Resource Directory.

Special Angels

Laura Rice – You deserve top billing in the angel category. Your generosity with your time, and willingness to always say, " **Yes, we can do that,**" has meant more to me that you can imagine. Countless times over the years that we have worked together, you have squeezed me into your schedule even though it was packed. Thank you for all your help on this book, and for being such a dear friend.

Mickey Schlatter, another angel. Thank you for saying, "yes" to my call for help. It made this project so much easier, to know I could depend on your editing expertise. I'm sure it turned out to be a bigger project than you anticipated, but you haven't complained. Thank you for that. As a bonus to me, you have become a warm and loving friend. I have truly enjoyed our time working and laughing together. I trust that our friendship will not end with this book.

Chirayu Borooah, one of the busiest men on the planet, and yet you were so kind and generous to **offer to read my manuscript.** I truly hope that it did not require a great deal more time than you had calculated in the beginning. Your suggestions of word changes, and sentence restructuring have been extremely valuable. You have contributed greatly to making this a better book. Thank you very much.

Karen Schuman, a friend for many years, Thank you for your help in obtaining copyright permission, for getting me the best prices possible and for your loving support.

H.D. Wilbanks, a very special angel. Thank you for taking a chance on me, and my Face-Saver Pillow. Your care and concern for my financial welfare went far beyond customer service. You are one of the exceptional people, who is never tuned into WIIFM (What's In It For Me). You are a true gentleman, with a level of integrity that, unfortunately, is rare.

Thank you for your valuable advice, incredibly honestly, and support.

Supporting Friends

Karen Mack, Thank you for your eternal words of encouragement and valuable feedback on everything. It means so much to have a prompt response when one is agonizing over a decision, and you're always there. You are my special "child."

Barby Genglebach, a long time, dear friend, and one is who always there for me. Thank you for your valuable feedback when I was searching for a book title, and your support in general.

Ondine Fortune, one of the busiest ladies I know, and yet you always make time for me. Thank you for helping me select a title, and thank you for rescuing me from the jaws of the **AMG sharks.**

June Samuelson, a friend forever. Thanks for helping with a title, for caring enough to ask, and then actually listening. Blessings.

A NOTE OF SPECIAL THANKS to the loving and compatible crew who pulled this all together.

Kathi Dunn, Dunn+Associates, for your magnificent artistry on the cover. You're the best!

Mary Jo Jirik, Dunn+Associates, for pleasantly keeping us on time.

Susan Kendrick, Susan Kendrick Writing, for your creative writing and keen observations.

Ted Goff, Cartoonist, for your warmth and great sense of humor. I needed some laughter.

John Williams, Guardian Printers, for your expertise in printing, and the education.

Fidel Bell, Embassy Media, for your warm and friendly cooperation, and great advice!

And, of course, *Laura Rice, Mickey Schlatter,* and *Chirayru Booroh.* Thank you all!

If I have left someone out, and I probably have, please accept my sincere apologies. As embarrassing as it is to have to admit this, I am currently suffering from temporary "sleep deprivation."

Introduction

Restful sleep is elusive for many people on a regular basis, especially women, but not exclusively women. The National Sleep Foundation reports that their surveys reveal 60 percent of adults have sleep problems a few nights a week. In addition, more than 40 percent of adults experience daytime sleepiness severe enough to interfere with their daily activities, at least a few days a week, or more.

Sleep is one of the most important factors in good health, mental clarity and emotional stability. Strangely enough, it seems when circumstances require that we call forth all of the above, sleep is the first thing that goes out the window.

This book was conceived to impress upon my clients and readers the absolute importance of sufficient sleep in their quest for beauty, health and anti-aging. It is crucial if you want radiant skin, with good elasticity, toned muscles and a stress-free countenance. It is also crucial for high self-esteem, self-confidence, vitality and energy. However, the more research I did on sleep, the more profound the subject became.

Being tired seems to be an epidemic in this country, and is getting worse, not better. Most of us have been too busy trying to "catch up", because we're so far behind, because we're so tired, that sufficient sleep has been totally neglected. I fully realize when you're running behind, it seems impossible to consider getting more sleep, but it is undoubtedly the most sensible thing to do.

Fatigue makes us feel overwhelmed in all areas of our life. I'm sure the statistics would be almost unbelievable if we could actually calculate the number of arguments between families, friends and co-workers that are caused by at least one side being overly tired.

Sleep deprivation is being attributed to all kinds of emotional, physical, and social problems in today's society. Uncontrolled anger, stress, low self-esteem, diminished libido, depression, pessimism/negativity, road rage, short fuses in general, poor work performance, poor memory, and many other maladies too numerous to mention can usually be traced back to lack of sleep.

Dr. James Maas, professor of psychology at Cornell University, and author of "Power Sleep", tells us that sleep deprivation actually shortens your life. He states that numerous studies show that sufficient sleep reduces the risk of heart attacks, immune disorders, and diabetes.

Dr. William C. Dement, M.D., Ph.D. is the world's leading authority on sleep, sleep deprivation, and the diagnosis and treatment of sleep disorders. In fact, he founded the first sleep disorder center at Stanford University in 1970, and launched the American Sleep Disorder Center in 1975. In his outstanding book "The Promise of Sleep," he makes the profound statements. "Healthful sleep has been empirically proven to be *the single most important factor in predicting longevity,* more influential than diet, exercise, or heredity. And yet, we are a sleep-sick society, ignorant of the facts of sleep – and the price of sleep deprivation."

According to research by the National Sleep Foundation, at least 40 million Americans suffer from some kind of sleep disorder, yet more than 60 percent of adults have never been asked about the quality of their sleep by a physician, and fewer than 20 percent even initiated a discussion.

The director of the National Center on Sleep Disorders Research, Dr. Carl E. Hunt, puts the number of problem sleepers at around 70 million. About half of this number have actual sleep disorders, and the others have a lifestyle that creates sleep problems.

We take in too much caffeine, sugar, alcohol; watch too much mindless television, and surf the net, so we don't get sufficient, regular exercise.

Yet, we still expect our bodies and minds to carry us through long hours of work and stressful commuting, as well as handling the demands of family responsibilities.

Sleep deprivation seems to be a totally neglected and accepted way of life. Even much of the medical community has ignored it. Many authorities are now calling it a national epidemic, and a serious public-health risk.

Even obesity can be contributed to sleep deprivation, and obesity is a major health risk. Research indicates that the later you stay up at night, the more you have a tendency to over-eat. Even if you don't stay up late, trying to maintain a diet of reduced calories is much more difficult when you're tired.

Perhaps even more dramatic statistics come from the National Sleep Foundation on the number of auto accidents caused by sleepy drivers. They report that fatigue contributes to more than *100,000* police-reported highway crashes, causing 71,000 injuries and 1,500 deaths each year in the United States alone.

How many people do you approach each day, or approach you with the question, "How are you?" How often do you hear, or respond, "Tired!" It's something to think about.

I trust the information in this book will educate you on the serious importance of sufficient sleep. I also sincerely hope you will be inspired and motivated to find your own perfect solution, and rearrange your life, so that you are no longer one of the walking, working and eating tired.

I urge you to do whatever is possible, and beyond what you thought was possible, in order to enjoy your own beauty/power sleep. It will change your life. You'll find that you will greet each new day with the energy of a sunrise, and the enthusiasm of a child.

"The sun does not awake as soon as I,
to greet the fair adventure of tomorrow."

William Shakespeare

CHAPTER 1

ࡇࡇ

What
Is
Sleep?

ࡇࡇ

"Sleep is a sort of innocence and purification.
Blessed is He who gave it to us.
Sleep is the sure and faithful companion of life.
Our daily healer and counselor."

Henri Frederic Amiel
Swiss Critic
1821 – 1881

Many people are puzzled about sleep. Exactly what is it? Why do we need it? Why are we healthier, happier and more productive with it, and irritable, unhealthy, and incompetent without it? What is this mysterious thing that we engage in almost one third of our life, and yet know so little about?

Sleep is an interesting and very complex subject. Most of us never give any thought to what sleep is, until we can't sleep. I thought it was a simple, basic biological process, which is part of our rhythmical pattern of life, which helps us move from day into night, and back again. It is this, but far more.

In Dr. William Dement's book, "The Promise of Sleep," he talks about sleep being a perpetual wall between the conscious mind and the outside world, and yet that wall is immediately reversible, as the sleeper can be awakened by noise.

Even though we may think that nothing is happening while we sleep, research indicates that quite a bit is going on. There are all kinds of brain activities and bodily functions in process.

Since I'm not a doctor or a sleep research scientist, I'm not qualified to even attempt to enlighten you on all the scientific facts about sleep. However, it is a fascinating subject, and if you want to delve into it more scientifically, I highly recommend you read "The Promise of Sleep" by Dr. William Dement and "Power Sleep" by Dr. James Maas.

Since our bodies are governed by internal biological clocks, I found the research done over twenty-five years ago by Dr. Franz Halberg and Dr. Daniel Kripke very interesting. They discovered that these biological clocks control all sorts of bodily functions other than sleep, such as appetite, emotional moods, body temperature, hormones, etc. However, what was especially interesting to me is our circadian rhythm. Did you realize if you could remove yourself from the outside world, and allow your body to "run free," that it would probably operate on a twenty-five hour cycle rather than a twenty-four hour cycle? We have entrained ourselves to the twenty-four hour cycle of our solar system and our social environment.

We actually have two basic, but completely different kinds of sleep, NREM (non-REM), and REM (Rapid Eye Movement).

There are very distinct patterns of brain waves in the different types and stages of sleep. You go through four stages of NREM sleep, then slip back into two of the NREM stages, and from there, move into REM sleep, which is when you dream.

Sleep begins with NREM. This is when your brain waves begin to slow down. Your body becomes quiet, as your muscles relax, your heart rate decreases, breathing slows down, and your body temperature drops. You are now in Stage 1 of your NREM sleep. This will last for a very short period of time, perhaps only five to ten minutes.

Then you move into Stage 2 of NREM sleep. This is still considered a light sleep stage. You can be awakened easily, but you will realize that you have been asleep. You are normally in this stage of sleep for approximately ten minutes.

Stage 3 is when you move into a deeper sleep,

and Stage 4 is when you move into your deepest stage of sleep. Your body functions slow down even more, with slower breathing and heart rate, blood pressure drops, and your muscles are extremely relaxed. Your mind and senses are also completely relaxed, and if you're awakened during this period of sleep, you will feel very groggy and perhaps even disoriented.

After being in Stage 4 sleep, for perhaps, thirty minutes, you will move back into Stage 3 and then Stage 2, and then proceed directly to your REM stage.

REM sleep is when your eyes dart back and forth beneath your lids. REM sleep starts out in short cycles – five to ten minutes. Then you move back into NREM sleep, but to stages 3 and 4 only. You repeat this process, throughout the night, with your REM sleep lasting longer with each cycle, perhaps as long as twenty to forty minutes.

REM sleep is when you do your dreaming. We experience rapid eye movement, as well as other physiological changes, such as a rise in body temperature, increased blood pressure, and respiratory changes. Males may experience an erection, and females may have a clitoral engorgement, but *our muscles are temporarily paralyzed*. I found this fascinating. This may explain why we sometimes have frustrations in our dreams about not being able to run or perform other activities that we feel we need to perform when our dreams seem to call for activity.

However, in reality, it is our Creator who once again is watching over us. This temporary paralysis protects us from danger or damage that we could possibly do to others, or ourselves, if we were to act out our dreams.

It's very important to experience NREM and REM sleep in order to awaken refreshed, renewed and rejuvenated. Researchers postulate that the purpose of the two kinds of sleep is that NREM sleep serves as a physical restoration, and REM repairs and reorganizes key brain connections and systems, which restores us mentally.

In Dr. William Dement's book, The Promise of Sleep, he discusses the fact that it has recently been discovered that the adult brain is able to grow new brain cells. This is in direct opposition to the long-standing dogma that after infancy, the brain does not generate new cells. Since we do grow new brain cells, and it is necessary to experience REM sleep in order to restore us mentally, it seems to confirm the importance of getting your REM sleep on a regular basis.

Don't you think it's time that we all showed a little more respect for this magnificent computerized system with which our Creator has blessed us, and start making sleep a priority in our lives?

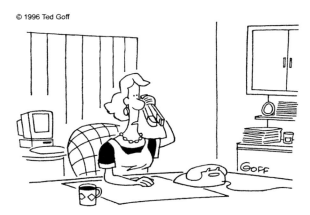

© 1996 Ted Goff

"I'm sorry I misdirected your call. I didn't get much sleep last night. Hello? Hello?"

CHAPTER 2

၉ဝ၂

How Much Sleep Do You Need?

ဢဝၑ

*"Take a rest.
A field that has rested
Gives a beautiful crop."*

Ovid
Roman Poet
1700

Although for most of your life, you have probably heard you need eight hours of sleep per night, many people need more. In fact, Dr. James Maas, author of "Power Sleep," feels that eight hours is not ideal, at least for peak performance. He suggests that the number is more like nine hours and twenty-five minutes for many people. Albert Einstein slept ten to twelve hours per night.

This amount of time devoted to sleep may seem unrealistic to you, but I urge you to love yourself enough to find out how much sleep you actually need, and then take positive steps to getting it. If you can't get it all, then at least get as close to it as humanly possible under your current circumstances.

In order to find out exactly how much sleep you really need, you have to set aside some time, perhaps a weekend or make it part of a vacation plan and sleep yourself out. Totally wipe out your sleep debt. Close the drapes and turn off the phone. Tell the rest of the family to awaken you only in case of an emergency. I mean a true emergency -- like a fire -- not because someone can't find a baseball bat, a blue sweater, or needs a ride to the mall. Don't set an alarm clock, physically or mentally. A very wise person said, "There is no hope for a civilization which starts each day to the sound of an alarm clock" Author unknown. I concur completely.

After you have eliminated your sleep debt, then you need to repeat this process of allowing yourself to sleep until you awaken naturally. If you continue to sleep nine hours each day, then you probably need nine hours of sleep. If you awaken and feel refreshed after eight or eight and a half, this is probably your requirement.

It would be a good idea for everyone in the

family to follow the program. Then when it's clear about the amount of sleep each family member requires, hopefully those who need less sleep will be more considerate about noise and needs, in order to accommodate the sleepers.

It is usually more difficult to find the time to "sleep in" an extra thirty minutes than it is to get to bed earlier. Therefore, make a sincere attempt at getting to bed just a little earlier, even if you have to start with ten or fifteen minutes. Once again, I ask you to analyze your time management. Was the fifteen minutes you spent on the phone with a friend complaining about the cost of gasoline, or the actions of the current administration really worth it? If you aren't going to take positive actions to correct a situation with which you're unhappy, then don't waste your time complaining about it. Your sleep is more important!

I fully realize some people are convinced they can function very well on six or seven hours sleep per night, and perhaps they can. We are all biological individuals. If you can truly manage this, and are not ignoring the symptoms of sleep deprivation, then I must admit, I'm a bit envious. I would absolutely love to have a few more productive hours each day. However, notice I said "productive."

I sometimes wonder if these "sleepless wonders" have ever taken the time to analyze whether or not they actually feel rested. It is easy, and really quite normal to be functioning on either stress or excitement, and think you're rested. If this is the case, believe me when I tell you, it will eventually take its toll.

There is an incredible amount of reliable research that indicates sleep deprivation, for whatever reason, definitely accelerates aging, and all the aggravations and maladies that come with it.

Sleep deprivation causes poor brain function. Some of the worst accidents recorded in history have been traced back to lack of sleep. Three-Mile Island, Exxon Valdez, and Chernobyl are all tragic examples of sleep deprivation, and there are a host of others that did not receive so much publicity.

Don't wait until something tragic happens in your life before you take steps to get the amount of sleep you really need.

༄༅

CHAPTER 3

The Magic Of Mind Control

ཞ༅

"Sleep is the best cure for waking troubles."

Cervantes, from Don Quixote
Spanish Novelist
1547– 1616

Our main objective at hand is sound, peaceful, and rejuvenating sleep. However, controlling our minds, our thoughts and feelings, is of utmost importance in achieving everything we want in life. It is crucial in handling stress and anxiety, two major sleep thieves. Mind control is always easier said than done, but well worth the effort necessary to accomplish it. In fact, I truly believe that learning to control your thoughts, feelings and beliefs, is the *most important asset that you can develop.* The research is indisputable that what we think about we manifest in our lives, or as many of my most valued mentors teach, "What we think about, we become."

All great thinkers, teachers and philosophers, past and present, have endeavored to enlighten us on the incredible power of our minds, and the importance of controlling our thoughts. Even though we may have heard this many times, it is not an easy discipline to incorporate into our busy lives, and especially if one is tired from lack of sleep. Most of the time one's mind is so full of present and urgent responsibilities, it seems impossible to quiet it long enough to get control over our thoughts. However, this is exactly what we must do in order to make positive changes in our life.

Because of this, I have found one of the greatest tools available in helping me to activate the power of my mind is subliminal message cassettes. They can accomplish what I cannot, by circumventing my conscious rejections, and going straight to my super, subconscious mind. Once your subconscious mind is convinced, you will find yourself feeling and acting in a manner that is in harmony with the new thought pattern. Then it will be easy for your conscious mind to agree. One of the great advantages of using the subliminal cassettes is that you can accomplish this without the stress and strain of trying to find the time to do it. You just listen.

If you experience insomnia, even periodically, or want to change your attitude about your eating and exercise habits, or increase your self-esteem/self-confidence, this is definitely an avenue you should investigate. For you who may not be familiar with subliminal tapes, we have provided an in-depth explanation in the appendix.

Try to avoid late telephone calls.

Even if calls are from friends and loved ones, conversation is stimulating, and will activate your mind. The results are even worse if the conversation involves something that is exciting or depressing.

Don't surf the net until it's time to turn out the lights.

This may be a boring or stimulating experience, but either way it has a tendency to hamper wind-down capabilities.

Avoid television just before bed.

It is more difficult to quiet your mind if you've been watching TV. Read something inspirational that will relax your mind. It's even better if you play a peaceful subliminal tape while you read. There's an old Indian saying — "A busy mind is a sick mind — a quiet mind is a healthy mind, and a still mind is a Divine Mind."

Meditation is best thing to do just before you get into bed.

Prayer and meditation are different. I feel it's very important to pray, but it is just as important to listen. If we are always doing all the talking, as we do in prayer, we can't hear the messages the Universe, or God is sending us. These messages may be the answers you need to eliminate the anxiety that quite often keeps people awake at night. Meditation is the key that opens the door to your Higher Self, your Divine Mind. It is not easy to learn to quiet one's mind to the point of not thinking, but once you learn to do so, the rewards are magnificent. Many people do not understand how the Divine Mind talks to us. Answers come to us in the form of a feeling, or an intuition. You ask to be shown the right way to do something, or an answer for a particular situation. Then you quiet your mind, knowing and believing the answer is on its way to you. Quietly wait with great expectation, and it will come. Maybe not in the same meditation session, but soon the answer will just pop into your head, or you'll have a strong feeling about what to do, and be comfortable with the decision. The mind is like a muscle, and it must be exercised regularly, in the way you want it to work for desired results, so stay with it.

Waking up in the middle of the night is not always a bad thing.

This may be when your Divine Mind in sending you the answer. Sometimes the most perfect solutions to problems and situations come to us in the middle of the night. Be sure that you keep a pen and pad at your bedside, jot down the thought, thank God for the answer, and then go back to sleep. Some people tell me that they turn on a small light. I prefer to jot the thought or answer down in the dark, as light awakens me instantly. It may not be the most perfect penmanship, but I can always read it well enough to understand the answer or idea the next morning.

Count Your Blessings!

This is one of my favorite ways to relax my mind. As the song lyrics go, "When I feel worried, and I can't sleep, I count my blessings instead of sheep, and I fall asleep counting my blessings."

When I say count your blessings, I mean *all of them.* Your body is the temple of your soul, and you should be incredibly grateful for the magnificence of it. Do an entire "organ recital", start with your toes, wiggle them, and be grateful that you can do this. Stretch your feet, and be grateful that you can do this. Circle your ankles, and be grateful that you can do this. Go through your entire body, acknowledge each part, i.e. your heart, your lungs, your glands, your blood, your eyes, ears, etc. If you happen to have something in your body that is currently not functioning to its highest level, bless it anyway. Blessing it will help it heal, complaining or cursing it, will keep it in a state of disease. By the way, don't forget your magnificent mind, your incredible brain, and the ability to learn and to grow.

When you finish with yourself, go through your family, friends, neighbors, and business associates. Find something about each one of them for which you can be grateful.

Give thanks for the rights and privileges you enjoy living in this great country, and list each one of them in your mind.

Go through your possessions, your home, your furniture, your appliances, your artwork, your accessories, your clothes, your jewelry, and anything else you cherish. It's endless!

There is nothing more uplifting, relaxing, and rewarding than counting your blessings.

Count your breaths.

This is another good way to turn off your mind. Concentrate on each breath and be grateful you can breathe freely. As you inhale, take in as much air as you can. Then exhale as slowly as possible. You will have a tendency to want to let all the air out at once. Do not do this. Controlling your exhaling will fatigue you, and before long you'll find you're very tired. It's also an excellent idea to tell yourself that as you inhale, that you're inhaling qualities you want to experience, and exhaling qualities you want to eliminate in your life. For instance, you might tell yourself as you inhale that you're bringing into your life peace, productivity, prosperity, confidence, health, and other blessings. As you exhale, you can tell yourself you're eliminating tension, anxiety, procrastination, poverty, or lack of any kind. This exercise will not only help you get to sleep, but it will program your super conscious mind to work in the way you want it to work throughout the night – since it never sleeps.

CHAPTER 4

༺ৡৡ༻

Seeking Solutions For Soothing Sleep

༺ৡৡ༻

"If my dear, you seek to slumber –
Count of stars an endless number
If you still continue wakeful,
Count the drops that make a lake full
Then is vigilance yet above you,
Count the times I love you,
And if slumber still repels you,
Count the times I did not tell you."

Franklin Pierce Adams
U.S. Author/Columnist
1881 – 1960

The Bible teaches, "Ask, and you shall receive. Seek and you shall find. Knock and it shall be opened unto you."

I trust that at least some of the following ideas will provide the help you are seeking to solve your sleep challenges. If not, I can only suggest that you ask a Higher Power for help, and perhaps do that anyway.

Create good sleep habits.

This probably sounds like a mantra that you've heard over and over again. However, it is step one in your journey to better sleep. Our bodies LOVE habit. Therefore, make it a priority to go to bed at a regular time, and get up at a regular time, even on weekends. It takes about 21 days to develop a habit, so give it time. If you maintain a hectic schedule where you have to travel, have late meetings, etc., do the best you can until you have a window of time to implement this. However, make this a goal, and don't postpone it indefinitely.

Develop basic bed behavior.

Use your bed for sleep and sex only. I'm sure Groucho Marx would disagree with this. He has been quoted as saying "Anything that can't be done in bed isn't worth doing at all." However, sleep experts tell us not to read, do paper work, watch TV, or eat in bed. Do all of these things in a chair. I talk to people frequently who tell me reading in bed helps them fall asleep, and if they have to get up and move to the bed, this activity wakes them up. If this is your experience, my advice is "read in bed." I do encourage you to be judicious about what you read though. Please make it something pleasant and quieting, no contracts, sales reports or newspapers.

Keep your bedroom neat and uncluttered.

A cluttered environment creates a cluttered mind, and that is not conducive to sleep. Learn to put things away as you finish with them. It isn't as difficult as it may sound. Hang up your clothes or put them in the hamper. As I mentioned above, it takes only about 21 days to create a new habit. Throwing your clothes on a chair, the bed or the floor is simply a bad habit.

If you have a reading chair in your bedroom, as I do, you know how easy it is to accumulate stacks of partially read books, magazines and articles. This needs to be an area of constant monitoring. Otherwise, it can get out of control, and you have a cluttered mess in your bedroom.

If at all possible, avoid having a desk or worktable in your bedroom. I've done this and know first-hand how destructive this can be to a restful sleep. If your current situation requires that you use your bedroom for work activities, then cover the work area before you go to bed. You might buy a nice pale blue sheet and drape it over your desk or table. At least you won't see all the work that needs to be done if you have to make a trip to the bathroom in the middle of the night.

In Chapter 6, *Create A Cozy Cocoon*, you'll find suggestions for making your bedroom a very special place for sleep and other sensual things.

Keep your bedroom relatively dark.

This may seem like a big order, if you have outside security lights, live on a well-lighted street, or in an apartment complex. These are all challenges that we face living in a metropolitan area. If you live in the country, or at least in a suburban area, these requisites will be easier to manage. You may find that you have to change your window coverings to a heavier drape or different type blind. If these suggestions are not feasible, how about wearing loose fitting eye shields, or lay a soft (preferably dark) cloth over your eyes. I find this works very well, as it's easy to remove if you need to do so, and doesn't leave lines on your face, as eye shields will do if they fit too tight.

Covering your eyes is sometimes the only solution if you're a houseguest or staying in a hotel, so keep this in mind when you pack your bags.

I feel little blue night-lights make it easiest to maneuver around in the middle of the night, without giving your eyes so much light that it wakes you up. Your eyes make a huge adjustment to light after being in the dark for several hours. You'll find the standard 5-7 watt nightlight, even though it seems dim when you go to bed, will appear rather bright in the middle of the night. If you're already having trouble sleeping, this may be just enough light to do you in for several hours more.

Keep your bedroom cool.

This enhances sleep more than one would imagine. Of course, this solution will vary depending on your geographical location and change from season to season. It is a general consensus that sleeping in a room approximately 65° F is ideal. It is far better to sleep in a cooler room, and use an electric blanket, than to keep your room warm. In fact, in the winter, an electric blanket is beneficial in many ways. If you find it difficult to get out of bed when the room is cold, make sure you put your wake-up clothes (sweats, robe, etc.) under the top cover. They will be so warm and cozy, that you'll pull them on with joy, and won't dread getting out of a cozy bed. Well, maybe a little, but warmed clothes makes it much easier.

There are a lot of good things to be said for electric blankets. They give you warmth, without weight. There is something very comforting about crawling into a warmed bed after a hectic day. As they say, "My day was so stressful, I'm going to go home, go to bed, and turn my electric blanket up to Mother."

Sleeping in a cool room is great, but being cold can keep sleep at bay. Sometimes you may wake up in a fetal position, which I guess isn't all that bad. However, if you're pulled tightly into this position, because you're cold, you are probably closing off your circulation, which isn't good. It seems if our feet are warm, we feel warm all over. For that reason, I understand that some companies are making electric blankets now with stronger heating elements in the lower area, in order to keep feet cozy.

Keep your bedroom quiet.

This is something that we can take complete control of inside our home. It may require some major family adjustments, but it can, and should be done. Most people "live too loud." Noise pollution has become a major factor in our lives, and surprisingly, many people don't even notice that it has happened. Televisions and stereos blare, so families have to yell at each other in order to be heard. People yell to each other from room to room rather than walking into the room and talking. You might like to create a "quiet hour" before bedtime. Turn everything down, and talk quietly to each other. It might even be fun to sort of "whisper." Take note of how much calmer you feel in this environment.

Years ago, I went to a dentist whose office environment was so peaceful and quiet that it totally calmed my nerves about the root canal I was about to endure. Everyone from the receptionist, to the nurse and the dentist himself, spoke in a calm, quiet tone of voice. One really had to listen, in order to hear, and that certainly would not be a bad policy for families to implement.

Other noise polluters from the inside are ticking clocks. Many battery operated clocks tick loud enough to interfere with sleep. Remove them. Clock watching will only enhance your anxiety about not being able to sleep, but if you want a clock near your bed, get an electric one, or put a pillow over your battery clock so you don't hear it tick. If you use an electric clock and it has a bright illuminating light, cover it.

The next little noise polluters may be the most painful to remove, and the majority of you will probably opt to live with them. *Pets in the bedroom.* Recently on the television show, Good Morning America, it was brought out that **96%** of the people surveyed admitted that pets who slept either in the bedroom, or in the bed with them, disturbed their sleep. However, almost everyone decided not to make any changes in this area. Now I can totally relate to not only the desire of wanting your VIP to sleep in your bed, but also to the incredible nightly sleep disturbance that a loveable, loyal and "member of the family" pet can inflict. Therefore, I will not criticize or be judgmental if you decide to "live with it." However, I would like to encourage you who may be thinking of getting a new pet, *not to allow them to sleep with you.* Your pet will feel just as loved and happy in his/her own little sleeping area, if this is all he/she knows. Older pets sometimes develop problems, just like older people. They may start to snore, have breathing problems, sleep more restlessly. This is usually not dangerous to the pet, but it certainly can disturb your sleep. You will be the only one who is sleep deprived. After all, napping during the day is one of the perks of being a pet.

Noise from the outside is not usually as easy to control. If it comes from neighbors, perhaps you could have a calm, friendly conversation about the problem, and see if you can reach some kind of a compromise. If it's comes from other factors, that you cannot control or change, you might try using a quiet fan, perhaps on low. The consistent hum will be beneficial in lulling you to sleep. You could also consider using other white-noise assistance, such as environmental tapes, or an actual white-noise machine, which will close out uncontrollable noises like crickets, street traffic, and other intrusions. Earplugs seem to have improved, so perhaps this is something for consideration, as well.

Now that we've addressed some of the environmental challenges that hamper sleep, let's see what we can do to provide you with additional solutions for soothing sleep.

Avoid caffeine before bed.

In fact, if you must indulge, it is better to do so before noon. This doesn't apply to just coffee, but tea, colas, and any kind of chocolate, including chocolate milk. It is an undisputed fact that caffeine has a tendency to keep people awake. In fact, many people medicate their fatigue during the day with caffeine, creating an unending cycle of sleepless nights and drowsy days.

Avoid alcohol before bed.

This does not mean that you cannot have a relaxing glass of wine with dinner, but it does mean that a nightcap is not recommended. Many people feel if they have a drink before they go to bed that it will help them sleep. It indeed may help them fall asleep faster, but it will definitely interfere with the quality of both their NREM and REM sleep. As you may remember, we discussed earlier the importance of getting both types of sleep to restore the body and repair brain functions. There is something else you should be aware of, and that is the danger of drinking alcohol at any time when you're sleep deprived. Sleep deprivation greatly magnifies the effects of alcohol, and you could find yourself drunk on one drink.

Eating right before bed has always been a bad habit.

If your stomach is full when you go to sleep, your body has to work at digesting the food, and sending it to the right channels, rather than repairing and rebuilding your cells, which is it's normal function during the sleep process. This habit is also a predictable path to obesity.

A full stomach can keep you awake at night, particularly if you were careless about what you ate. This is particularly true if you eat foods that are high in sugar, spices or heavy proteins. However, it is also impossible to sleep if you're actually hungry, and your blood sugar is too low. Therefore, try to eat about an hour before bedtime. Make wise choices about what you eat, and eat only enough to satisfy your hunger. We have covered bedtime food and drink choices, as well as herbs and supplements in Chapter 5.

Drink water, by all means, drink water, but drink it 30 to 45 minutes prior to bedtime.

Drinking sufficient water is a crucial component for health and beauty, following closely behind sufficient sleep. Seventy-five percent of Americans are chronically dehydrated. Of this group, thirty-seven percent have developed such a weak thirst mechanism, that they mistake thirst for hunger. Maybe you don't actually need a bedtime snack; maybe you just need a glass or two of water. Water is so critical, because our body contains so much water – approximately 40-50 quarts of water. Blood is 83% water, muscles are 75% water, *your brain is 74% water,* and your bones contain about 22% water. It also lubricates your joints, keeps your tissues from sticking together, keeps your blood from becoming thick, so your heart doesn't have to work so hard at pumping it. It's essential for every function.

The best time to drink water is early in the morning when your stomach is empty. This facilitates the removal of toxins that have collected in your kidneys while you were sleeping. Do not drink water *with your food; it dilutes your digestive enzymes.* Drink water 10-15 minutes prior to a meal. If you have been drinking water with your meals, and this seems like an impossible adjustment, you will be pleasantly surprised to find that drinking water before a meal eliminates most of your thirst during a meal. If you find that you cannot enjoy your meal without a drink of water, then have a small sip. It's best to wait about 2-3 hours after a meal before you start drinking water again. Of course, this depends somewhat on what you've eaten. Heavy proteins, like red meat, require about 3 hours for proper digestion, fish takes only about 2 hours, and a vegetarian meal could even be less.

If you drink water just before bed, you will

undoubtedly have to answer a call from nature before it's time to get up. This trip to the bathroom may be just enough activity to awaken you to the point where you have trouble going back to sleep. If you're taking a sleep aid, such as herbs, and/or drinking herbal tea, do it about 30 minutes before you're ready to go to bed, and then make one last trip to the bathroom whether you feel you need it or not. This may keep you in bed all night.

Exercise regularly, but not just before bed.

We are referring to intense or aerobic exercise, not gentle stretching, or yoga type moves. Stretching is quite often extremely beneficial in helping one de-stress, and get a good night's rest. Of course, sexual exercise certainly falls into the category of intense/aerobic exercise, but hopefully, and ideally the culmination of the activity will provide both partners with an orgasm, which is very sleep inducing for most people.

Try to do your regular workouts early in the day. There are numerous benefits to this, not the least of which is that you will have a better chance of actually getting it done. Once the day gets in gear, it is often quite difficult to find the opportunity to stop it long enough to workout.

CHAPTER 5

၆ၜ

Healthy Natural Sleep Aids

ಔಲ್

"Health is the first Muse.
Sleep is the condition to produce it."

Ralph Waldo Emerson
U.S. Essayist and Poet
1803 – 1882

In my opinion, it is always desirable to use natural substances over drugs for sleep inducement, or anything else, as far as that goes. I highly recommend that you avoid sleeping pills of any kind unless your doctor is adamant about your use of them. Even over the counter sleeping pills are undesirable.

Herbs are natural substances, but *should not be used indiscriminately.* Read labels, ask for guidance from your health store nutritionist, pharmacist, or health care provider, and *always check with your doctor if you're taking medications.*

Some of the most common and effective herbal remedies are as follows:

SLEEP – an herbal formula from Solaray, is a combination of Valerian, Hops, Skullcap, Passion Flower and other sleep inducing herbs. If you cannot find this, you may want to try just a Hops and Valerian combination. However, my experience has been that the SLEEP formula is more desirable. These herbal formulas seem to work well, just taking one or two 30 minutes before bedtime.

Chamomile Tea – This tea calms the digestive system, as well as the mind. A wonderful tea to drink after dinner or before bed.

Bed Time Tea is a blend of a variety of comforting herbs and has become an important part of my bedtime ritual. It contains Chamomile Flowers, Lemon Grass, Tilia Flowers, Spearmint Leaves, Passionflower Leaves, as well as other fruits and flowers.

Passionflower and Lemon Balm are other teas that you may like to use.

Make sure that any tea you drink is *herbal, and caffeine free.* Many people are very excited about the health benefits of green tea, but they don't consider that unless tea is caffeine free, your chances of sound sleep are minimal.

Kava – Although the herbs mentioned above do a very good job of calming anxiety, Kava seems to be the master for this sleep thief, which is a major cause of insomnia. Anxiety is particularly associated with the type of sleep deprivation that comes in the middle of the night, after 4-5 hours of sleep. If there is anxiety involved, it seems to be extremely difficult to turn off the mind and get back to sleep. If you are in a state of temporary anxiety in your life, it would be better to take ONE capsule before you go to bed, (do not mix with alcohol) rather than when you wake up in the middle of the night. This would be true of all sleep inducing herbs. Enzymatic Therapy® produces an excellent formula called KavaTone. *One note of caution concerning Kava.* Records of Kava's consumption date back to the 1600's, (sometimes referred to as Kava-Kava). South Pacific cultures have drunk concoctions of this plant for thousands of years. However, as in the use of any herbal or pharmaceutical medication, *it should not be abused.*

In my opinion, Kava has recently come under unfair attack due to bad publicity about *possibly* causing liver damage. According to a toxicology report issued in February 2002, Professor of Pharmacology and Toxicology, Dr. Donald P. Waller, PhD., of the University of Illinois, Chicago, states, "Kava has no scientifically established potential for causing liver damage when taken in appropriate doses."

The German studies that have caused them to ban Kava, did not take into consideration other factors such as using Kava with alcohol, and other prescription drugs. Even the FDA who is anything but kind and lenient where the natural supplement industry is concerned, stated in March 2002 that "liver damage appears to be rare," but consumers should be informed of this potential risk."

According to the American Botanical Council (ABC), a safe dosage for Kava is 300 mg of a standardized extract (70% kavalactones) daily. Do not take longer than four weeks at a time.

I would like to express my gratitude to "Let's Live," who provided the above statistical information and update on the Kava controversy.

Harold H. Bloomfield, M.D., an internationally respected psychiatrist, wrote an interesting book titled "Healing Anxiety with Herbs." In his book he states, "Kava is an intelligent choice for many people – it's safe and dependable, based on the latest scientific research."

Kava has been extremely successful in taming anxiety for many people, for many years, without harmful side effects. I for one would not like to be without it. I may take only one every few months, but always keep it on hand, and never abuse it.

However, if you have any concerns or are apprehensive about using KAVA, by all means check with your doctor.

If you have not used herbs in the past, and are wondering where to start, check our Resource Directory.

Melatonin is a natural hormone secreted by the pineal gland, which is located in the brain. It's production rises at night and falls during the day, which affects our sleep cycles. It is quite often used by middle-aged to elderly insomniacs, because the level of Melatonin declines with age. Most studies indicate that it is safe to use supplementation when levels are low. However, this should be checked, and you should understand that long-term effects, and ideal dosage are still being researched. I've talked with people who take it and love the results, but *do check with your doctor, or health practitioner.* I do not use it, as I find the herbs, and subliminal tapes work very well for me.

Magnificent   minerals are crucial supplements to induce a good night's sleep. Make sure that you're getting ample calcium and magnesium. We hear a lot about calcium. In fact, many people are almost obsessed with calcium. However, did you realize that calcium needs magnesium in order to assimilate into the body? When too much calcium is being consumed, in ratio to magnesium, the calcium will pull magnesium out of body parts in order to assimilate. This can cause all kinds of health problems, as well as sleep disorders, i.e., restless sleep, tension sleep and trouble sleeping in general. Peter Gillham, who is a clinical nutritionist, chemist and pioneer in the field of nutritional research, has developed a product called Natural Calm™. This is powdered magnesium, and works miracles in providing a calm, tension free, restful night's sleep. I use it with my Bed Time tea, and sleep with less tension that I ever thought was possible. Women going through menopause quite often have major sleep problems. The women that I have introduced to Natural Calm have only good results to report. It is also extremely helpful for women experiencing PMS anxiety. See Resource Directory for additional information.

Calcium, of course, is extremely important for sleep, bones, nerves and health in general. I do not mean to diminish its importance by the focus on magnesium. It's just that I feel we are inundated with information of taking sufficient calcium, and magnesium is sometimes overlooked.

Vitamin C, B-Complex and extra Pantothenic Acid are also very helpful in aiding sleep. Both Vitamin C and B-Complex work to nourish the nervous system, as well as give us a plethora of other health and beauty benefits.

If you find that you're having unpleasant dreams, or nightmares, as many Americans have since September 11, 2001 researchers have found that extra B-12, taken with B-Complex, is quite often very helpful. B-12 is generally more effective if you take it in sublingual form (under the tongue), rather than swallowing a tablet.

Bed time snack ideas: Snacks should be eaten about 45 minutes to an hour before you go to bed. This gives your digestive system a little time to work.

The amino acid tryptophan seems to have a sedative effect on many people. Foods that are high in tryptophan include yogurt (plain, not sugary fruit yogurts), turkey, peanut butter, and tuna. Also some high carbohydrate foods such as dates and figs contain tryptophan. However, I cannot recommend sugary foods before bed. I feel they raise the blood sugar level too high, too fast and whatever benefit comes from the tryptophan is lost. Some carbohydrates may work to induce sleep if they are complex carbohydrates, such as pasta, *non-sweetened* cereal and bread.

I would recommend that you stay with easy to digest, non-sweet snacks such as:

Plain low-fat yogurt. You can make it more interesting and nutritious by adding a tablespoon of raw sunflower seeds. This snack not only induces sleep, but also is fabulous for your skin. Keep in mind that I said *raw – not roasted and salted.* Raw seeds and nuts are delicious if kept in the freezer. This not only extends the shelf life, but also gives them a crunchy texture.

Warm milk – plain milk – not chocolate milk.

Brown rice. This is quite good cold, with plain yogurt. If you cook it early in the day, and keep it in the refrigerator it's ready for a snack without a lot of preparation.

Plain pasta would be acceptable, as well, but not with a spicy dressing.

Other protein foods that I use and recommend are liquid amino acid concentrates.

Amino Fuel® was recommended to me by a doctor to increase my protein intake. I don't eat huge amounts of food, and at the time was pretty much a vegetarian.

I am not by any means a true vegetarian, as I eat dairy all the time, and fish periodically. However, he felt it would be wise for me to get more protein, and suggested this as an avenue to do so. Liquid amino acid concentrates are quite often used by body builders, since they need such huge amounts of protein.

I prefer to use this if I wake up in the middle of the night, and feel my blood sugar has dropped. It is effective, and so much more convenient than eating regular food. The process of pulling out a dish, searching for a spoon, and eating food can really wake one up. If you have your own private bottle, you can just drink a few swallows, drink a little water, and you're back in bed. It is easy to digest, and will slowly raise your blood sugar, so you can get back to sleep.

Another protein supplement that enhances sleep is a product called **Calorad®.** Calorad has been around for 20 years, and has helped millions of people. Yet, I find that a lot of people are not familiar with it. It is actually a collagen supplement. Collagen is a natural protein that provides your body with structural support, and greatly improves muscle tone, skin tone and general connective tissue. If taken right before bed, on an *empty* stomach, not only will you sleep well, but it will also help build muscle and burn fat. When I was taking it at night, I noticed that it greatly improved my sleep, almost immediately. However, I also found that it was burning so much fat that I was losing weight, which I did not want to do. Therefore, I now take it in the morning, so I can get the benefits of the collagen, without the weight loss. If you want to sleep better, and lose weight, look into this.

Raw Apple Cider Vinegar mixed with water is another drink that is helpful for the 3:00 AM syndrome. Sometimes one's sleep cycle is interrupted by an acid/alkaline imbalance in the body. This mixture can quickly restore this balance. It's also wonderful to drink during the day to keep acidic crystals from forming which causes stiffness. It is also excellent for digestion, and appetite control.

Mix 1 teaspoon of RAW Apple Cider Vinegar with 8 ounces of pure water. Two popular brands are Hain® and Bragg™. These can be found in any good health store, and some super markets.

CHAPTER 6

༄་ཨ་

Creating

A

Cozy Cocoon

൲ൕ

"Dreams of the summer night!
Tell her, her lover keeps
Watch, while in slumbers light
She sleeps! My lady sleeps!"

Henry Wadsworth Longfellow
United States Poet
1807 – 1882

Two of the most important factors in creating the perfect bedroom is to make it feel safe and sensual. Start thinking of your bedroom as a very special personal retreat in your home. It should be a place for sleeping, relaxing, reflecting, meditation, and of course, romance. I realize this may seem idyllic to some of you, but I do hope you will be able to incorporate at least a few of these ideas. You may be able to start with only one or two, but it's a step in the right direction. We truly are a product of our environment, and if your sleep environment is cluttered, bright, busy and noisy, it will not be conducive to sleep or other sensuous activities.

Start with your lighting. One of my favorite inventions in our modern world is dimmers. I absolutely love them. They are marvelous for every room in the house, but especially important in bedrooms and bathrooms. The advantage is that when a bright light is necessary, it's available. If you cannot arrange to have dimmers installed, then have a lamp or two with low wattage, and use soft pink or ivory bulbs, so you can create the effect of a dimmer. Not only does this lighting set the stage for sleep and tranquility, it also sets the stage for romance and intimacy.

Another idea I really like for lighting is to use little Italian white lights in a large plant, a small tree or around the top of the room. Here again, the ideal situation would be to have them attached to a dimmer switch. They create a very charming, relaxing and sensuous atmosphere.

I truly love candles all over the house, but especially in the bedroom and bathroom. However, **please be very careful with candles.** Perhaps you can have one or two floating in a bowl of water, or a candle that is created in a bowl. I really think it's safest to keep candlesticks for the dining table. If you are not the type of person who is very judicious about candles, then don't even bring them into the bedroom. It's better to just use small lights.

Music is a sensual addition to the bedroom and bath area. It's ideal to have speakers placed in an obscure location, so you can keep the music very low, and yet audible. Keep in mind that you want this area to be calm, and relaxing. Be sure your choice of music reflects this mood. Listen to romantic songs and/or environmental selections.

The bed, of course, is the focal point of all bedroom activity. You should give lots of consideration to your bed. After all, hopefully, you're going to spend approximately one third of your life there.

You have to ignore advertising when you consider purchasing a mattress. There just isn't a one-size fits all. In fact, there may be a dramatic difference in mattress needs and comforts between you and your sleep partner. I can't imagine how people sleep on a very soft mattress, and others cannot imagine how I can sleep on such a firm mattress. If you have this conflict between you and your partner, you might consider buying two twin mattresses, one firm, and one soft. Use twin size bottom sheets, but use king size for the top sheet, blankets and comforter or bedspread. This way you can each have your preferred mattress, and still be under the same bedcovers.

Spend the most that your budget will allow for quality sheets. The higher the thread count, the better the quality. I know sheets and bedding can get outrageously expensive, but they add so much comfort and make you feel so luxurious. If you take proper care of them, they will last a long time. When you figure the price per night, it really isn't all that much.

Take a good look at your walls and see if they make you feel quiet and relaxed. Most people agree that a soft or off-white color for walls is relaxing. Also, pale blue and a soft green are wonderful colors for a bedroom. Warm ivory is very flattering to many skin tones. Just make sure that the colors are compatible with your personality. Making *you* feel peaceful and passionate should be your goal.

I've read that Joan Collins requests the wall color changed in the hotel suite where she will be staying, and they actually do it for her. She loves a soft peach, and feels it creates a warm glow in the room that resembles the same beneficial effects of candlelight.

After you have determined your preferred color, decorate the walls with only a few peaceful paintings, or special ones that bring you joy. Display photographs of people you love, and special occasions or vacations.

If possible, try to position your bed near a window that you can leave **partially** open at night. I'm a strong advocate of keeping your bedroom safe. Leaving a window wide open, unless you're on a second floor without a balcony access, is inviting trouble. This is true no matter how safe you think your neighborhood is. Statistics show that many women are raped in their own bedroom by an intruder who entered through an open window.

Keep your bedroom safe in other ways as well. Don't clutter walk areas with extension cords, shoes, clothes and other items you could trip over in the dark. Don't position hanging lamps over the bed. Also, don't arrange your bed to be near a bookcase or other furniture where items could fall on you in the event of an earthquake. You may not think about these things consciously when you're awake, but the subtle discomfort may be brought forth when you're in your alpha state.

While we're on the subject of safety, check the doors and windows in all areas of your home. Make sure that they are securely locked. When you're making your rounds, check to make sure the stove and electrical appliances are turned off. The idea is to put your mind at ease.

If you really want to create an ideal furniture arrangement, you might want to look into Feng Shui. This is the ancient Oriental art of placing furniture in your home to create balance and harmony. Some believe that the position of your bed can make or break a marriage. This may be a bit extreme, but certainly we all know that furniture placement, with or without Feng Shui, can make us comfortable or uncomfortable in a room.

Flowers in the bedroom add the ultimate touch of sensuality and romance. I feel there is nothing quite as romantic as soft white or cream roses in a bedroom. This is the crème de la crème of elegance, tranquility and romance.

Unfortunately fresh cut flowers require a considerable amount of daily care, if they are cared for properly. Therefore, you may have to leave fresh flowers for special weekends or occasions, and use a flowering plant in the bedroom. Another option would be to use only a single rose, or a bud vase of flowers. This can still give a feeling of romance and tranquillity without too much care.

Green plants are wonderful to have in the bedroom, as well. They not only add an attractive touch to the room, but they provide a source of oxygen.

These are only suggestions and enhancements that work for me. You must find your own path to your ideal bedroom. I only hope you will take the time to look at your current sleep environment, and ask yourself what you can do to make it more conducive to rest and relaxation.

If your budget does not allow you to buy new sheets, or fresh flowers, then just clear out the clutter and turn down the lights. This will be a start, and I believe you will feel so much better about yourself and your environment, that you will find a way to take the next steps.

Go through magazines and newspaper ads that may show a room or the placement of furniture that pleases you. Tear out the picture and put it up to remind yourself of how you want your room to look.

You can also go through furniture stores, or model homes are even better. Wonderful ideas can come to you through model home tours.

Also, watch Home & Garden Television (HGTV). Their programs provide a plethora of ideas on how to redo your space for a very small amount of money.

CHAPTER 7

ౡ౦ఞ

Sex and
Sleep
Deprivation

ౚ౦ఞ

*"An intellectual is a person
who's found one thing
that's more interesting than sex."*

Aldous Huxley
English Novelist
1894 – 1964

A wise man said, *"Sex is like money.   It
doesn't matter too much unless you don't have
enough."*   I suppose this could be said about a lot
of things in life that we consider necessities, or
even creature comforts.

We're not going to delve into a lot of
scientific research about sleep deprivation and sex
drive, as well as sexual performance. However, if

sexual performance is a major problem between you and your partner, a visit to a sleep research center is an intelligent decision.

It is rather simple to determine through a sleep pattern examination, whether the symptoms of male impotence is a psychological or physiological problem. Once this is accomplished, proper steps should be taken to correct it.

If a female partner is suffering from sexual performance, this should be attended to as well. Hormonal changes in the female body create all kinds of roadblocks to enjoyable sex, and should not be ignored. However, this is sometimes the case, since female problems are not as physically easy to detect, as male impotence.

My main reason for doing this chapter is to help people understand the connection between the sometimes ongoing, somewhat silent, destruction of great sex, and sleep deprivation.

The majority of the time, the downward spiral of a happy sex life has absolutely nothing to do with any type of serious sexual dysfunction.

It is far too often created by money problems, long work days, short attention spans, even shorter tempers, feelings of low self-esteem, high expectations, and *sleep deprivation.* In other words, a *Lifestyle Dysfunction.*

I'm not going to try to convince you that sleep will eliminate all of the above mentioned problems. However, I can tell you, unequivocally, sleep will help you to cope with these problems, and will quite often erase a lot of them over time. It may not take all that much time either.

If you're spending a considerable amount of money over what you're earning, needless to say, sleep won't take care of this situation. Nor will it handle long work days, but if you're thinking better and more productive, because you are getting sufficient sleep, perhaps your work days can be a little shorter.

Generally, women need a little more TLC when it comes to keeping their libido afloat than do men. Women need to feel that they're attractive and desirable. This is quite often determined by feeling rested and relaxed, as well as having a little time for personal care.

Men are blessed with all that great testosterone, which usually keeps them ready and willing, anytime, anywhere. It doesn't matter to a man if he has gained a few pounds, or if his hair hasn't been shampooed, but it might to a woman.

I don't mean to indicate that this is true of all women and all men, but usually this is pretty much the norm.

It is also important to point out that by nature, women seem to worry more than men, are lighter sleepers, and are quite often (but not always) the main caretakers of the children and the pets, as well as other household responsibilities. Therefore, they are quite often more tired than men. I see this role sharing changing, and I want to applaud the men who are making this happen.

Many men are also suffering from personal and social changes, which have affected their sex drive, as well as their sleep debt. There have been so many social changes concerning the male role over the past ten to fifteen years, that some men tell me they don't feel their role is as well defined as it once was at one time. This sometimes affects their self-esteem, which in turn can affect their sex drive.

The goal that I want to accomplish here is to get you to take a look at your lifestyle. Is it creating sleep deprivation? Is your sleep deprivation creating sexual deprivation? Is your sexual deprivation creating sleep deprivation? Quite often one will create the other, and you end up on an endless cycle. It is sometimes difficult to sleep well without sex, and difficult to have sex without sleep.

If your sleep partner says, "I'm just too tired to have sex tonight," it is probably very true, and has absolutely nothing to do with how much you are loved, or how much you are desired. If you're hearing this frequently, its time that you pay attention.

See what small changes can be made in your lifestyle to give you and your partner some quiet time together. Just restful, relaxed time, without a cloud of sexual expectancy hanging over you. Take a nap together. Enjoy each other, and recall the wonderful times you've had, and the love you feel for each other.

If possible, try to set some time aside on a weekend when business and family responsibilities won't have the intense time urgency that they do during the week. Just try this one weekend, and see how magnificent you feel, and how incredible you look!

It's even better if you can arrange to get away for the weekend. This is particularly important if you have children at home. Experience how much better you feel when you've had sufficient sleep, and your mind is relaxed. I think you'll be amazed at how quickly you'll find your lost libido.

If you're on a tight budget, try staying at home. If you have children, send them to a family member or friend for the weekend. Offer to reciprocate.

Turn off your phone!!! Order food in! Be totally involved in each other, but also be careful and intelligent.

"It is not economical to go to bed early to save the candles if the result is twins." *Chinese Proverb*

Beauty Sleep

*"I swear they are all beautiful.
Every one that sleeps is beautiful."*

Walt Whitman
American Poet
1819 – 1912

Looking for the Fountain of Youth? Try your bedroom!

Remember Briar Rose (Sleeping Beauty)? I'm not suggesting that you sleep for 100 years, but look what it did for her. A much younger man fell in love with her the moment he set eyes on her; they got married and lived happily ever after.

When it comes to beauty, sleep is highly underestimated. It's an amazing beauty aid. In fact, it's one of the most potent beauty contributors we have available. If sleep could be bottled and sold, it would outsell any product on the market today. Not only does it improve the quality and appearance of your skin, it also greatly improves muscle tone. As you know, muscle tone and youth are synonymous.

Sleep is when everything in your body repairs. It improves your vision, and makes your eyes sparkle. Because you're not fighting the pull of gravity your scalp gets more nourishment at night, which improves the health of your hair.

Posture plays an *extremely* important part in looking beautiful, youthful and confident at any age. It has been said that great posture can shave at least five years off your age visually, and also make you look as if you've lost five to ten pounds. However, if you're sleep deprived, chances are good that you have not had the energy to exercise regularly. If your muscles are weak and too tired to hold you up, you develop an old, haggard, and insecure appearance. This can become a habit so fast that it's terrifying. Not only does bad posture destroy your appearance (even if you're very young and otherwise beautiful), but it's harmful to your health in general.

When you have poor posture, you slump. When you do this you do not get proper oxygen into your lungs. Insufficient oxygen creates anaerobic cells in your body, which will create a whole host of health problems. This is a subject that is truly close to my heart, but too involved to go into in this book. If you want to learn more about this, I suggest that you read Tonita deRaye's book, "The Oxygen Answer." She provides medical statistics on cancer and anaerobic cells that are profound. Good posture fosters deep breathing, which increases oxygenation in your body.

Poor posture encourages back and neck problems. It also crowds your internal organs, and heaven knows gravity does a number on our organs, without the help of bad posture.

Vitality and high energy are both important to looking your best. I'm sure you have all known, or know of someone who impresses you as being ageless simply by their vitality and energy. One of the first people who comes to my mind is Art Linkletter, who celebrated his 90th birthday in July 2002. I consider him "my hero." He's beautiful in every aspect of life, and looks and acts 25-30 years younger than his chronological age. By the way, he sleeps 8-8½ hours per night. I love his comment, "You may not be able to turn back the clock, but you can certainly rewind it." It's very difficult to muster up vitality and energy, if you're suffering from sleep deprivation.

Sufficient sleep greatly improves our attitude about life, our ability to handle stress, our personality in general, and how we react to other people. If you don't believe this, watch how a cranky, irritable, irritating child is magically turned into a happy, joyful and loveable little angel after a nap, or a good night's sleep. As adults we may think we are controlling ourselves, but more often than not, our fatigue shows up in our attitude and abruptness, as well as our facial expressions.

Lack of sleep can destroy a well-meaning diet in a heartbeat. In fact, fatigue is probably one of the main reason why people fall off the diet wagon. Most dieters admit that they have a tendency to go overboard at night. This is usually because they are tired, and their enthusiasm toward their goals has diminished, because of this. The diet breakdown also quite often appears around Thursday. Why Thursday? It's coming close to the end of the work-week for many, and they just don't have the energy that they had starting out after the weekend. Getting proper sleep every night will quite possibly cure the Thursday syndrome.

If you're not getting the results you think you should have from your workouts, or if you just don't have the energy to do as much exercise as you would like – look at your sleep schedule. Sleep is often the missing link to fitness that most people never consider.

In doing research for this book, I learned that our muscles feel stiff and sore if we don't get sufficient Stage 4 sleep, which you may remember is your deep sleep stage. This is because our muscles heal and repair in Stage 4. Therefore, it's truly important, whether you have had a strenuous workout, or have just been using your muscles in your work, that you get deep sleep.

Are You Aging Your Face Every Time You Sleep?

As we mentioned at the beginning of this chapter, sleep is one of your most potent beauty aids. However, it you're sleeping improperly, it can actually be detrimental is some ways, and you need to make sure this does not happen to you.

Be aware of how you are sleeping, and make sure that your beauty sleep is not giving you morning nightmares. Sleeping on your face, will not only create lines and wrinkles in your skin, but it will breakdown your facial muscles, which are really quite small.

The human head is far heavier than most people realize. Most research puts head weight at 7-10 lbs., depending on the size and gender of the person. Now this may not seem like very much weight, but if you pick up a 7 or 10 pound weight, or even a good bookend, you may change your mind. Sleeping on your face is like sleeping with a weight resting on your face, and I doubt if you would knowingly do this. The Face-Saver Pillow® was designed specifically to protect your face from this kind of damage, because it curves around the outside of your face, and bears the weight of your head. It will also protect the financial investment that you make in your face. This is of particular importance if you invest in any kind of professional services, cosmetic surgery, or laser treatments.

Some people not only sleep on their face, but they also sleep with their hands under their face. This not only creates facial damage, but this position cuts off circulation in your hands. It also creates lines in your hands. All of this damage will show up as premature aging, which is totally unnecessary.

The same advice goes for your arms. Do not sleep on your arms. Try to get into the habit (and it can be created) of sleeping with your hands and arms outstretched, so you're not cutting off the circulation to this area.

Are you tense when you sleep? Have you ever taken the time to analyze whether you are or not? Do you have any idea how detrimental this sleep tension can be not only to your appearance, but also to your health, over the years? If you grind your teeth, if your body feels tight and stiff when you wake up, if your face looks tense in the morning, you are undoubtedly sleeping with tension.

Due to stress, some people sleep with their lips puckered. I discovered this the hard way – from personal experience. It creates ugly lines over the upper lip, which are very difficult to eliminate, as long as you continue this habit. One of the best aids for keeping this area of your face relaxed is to do mouth exercises. I'm a strong advocate of facial exercising, but *you must be extremely careful in the program you use, and make sure that the exercise you're performing is not creating lines and wrinkles in other areas of your face. This is absolutely crucial.* Many facial exercise programs on the market do just that. See the resource section for additional information on this.

You can also use a small facial vibrator to eliminate tension in your face. If you use a small vibrator, make sure that you're following the muscles in the right direction. Do not go against the muscle movement. If you are not familiar with facial muscles, see the Resource Directory in the back of this book, for a free diagram.

Many vibrators, even small ones, are too powerful to use directly on your face. I recommend covering the attachment with a soft, thick cloth, so you protect your skin from broken capillaries, and other damage. Preferably, use a velour/terrycloth towel, or something comparable. Start with just a few *seconds,* and work up to about 30-45 seconds. Try both low and high speeds to see which is more comfortable for your individual needs. By all means, follow directions on the unit, and *never use on swollen/inflamed areas, on veins or in the front of your neck.*

I find that a vibrator is particularly helpful for mouth tension, so I use it only in this area of my face, and on the back of the neck/shoulder area, which is another tension hot spot.

Use your sleep time to improve your hands,

nails and feet. After applying your moisturizer, apply white Vaseline and slip into cotton gloves and socks. This may take some adjusting, so if you can only handle this for a few hours to begin with, do it just a few hours, but the longer you stay with it, the easier it will be to sleep like this. If you find that you're waking up, then by all means, remove them. Your sleep is far more important. This is just a little beauty bonus, because you will wake up with satin smooth hands and feet.

If you sleep with a partner, I would suggest that you do this after the lights are out for the night, or completely skip it on special nights of lovemaking. It isn't something that has to be done every single night in order to bring you benefits. It's also difficult to do in the summer months when it's hot. Don't force yourself to do this, if you think it will interfere with your sleep. It just isn't worth it.

During sleep time your cells rejuvenate, your mind recuperates and your soul renews. Your entire being is dependent upon sleep for renewal. Don't sell yourself short by sleep deprivation. After all, you deserve to be the very best you can be, and there is no way you can accomplish this without sufficient sleep. Please take the time to determine how much sleep is sufficient for you, and then begin a program to reach this goal.

I'm sure I mentioned this earlier, but it's sort of a mantra with me, and I feel it's worth repeating. Sleep is our most powerful ally in our quest for beauty, health and anti-aging. There isn't any cream you can put on your face, any procedure you can do, or any supplement/medication you can ingest that can or will perform to its highest potential without sufficient sleep.

According to a recent survey by the National Sleep Foundation, 71% of the population said they would sleep more if they felt it would improve their appearance. Well, I have good news – *IT DOES!*

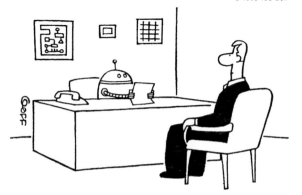

"What's this on your resume about
requiring food, water and sleep?"

CHAPTER 9

❧❧

Sleep For Success!

❧❧

*"It is a common experience that a problem
difficult at night is resolved
in the morning,
after the committee of sleep
has worked on it."*

John Steinbeck
U.S. Novelist (Nobel Prize 1962)
1902 – 1968

It doesn't matter whether you're an adventurous entrepreneur, climbing the corporate ladder, or somewhere in between, stress in business seems to be inevitable. There are problems to be solved, deadlines to meet and people to sell, to convince and appease.

Then there are those eternal decisions, decisions and decisions. This aspect of business affects men and women in every walk of life. This is true whether you're riding the stock market roller coaster, deciding on other investments, expanding your business, cutting back your business or changing jobs. The challenge of decision-making ranks pretty close to the top of the scale for sleep deprivation. This is unfortunate, as a good night's sleep greatly enhances one's ability to make wise decisions. I'm sure you have all heard the saying, "I want to sleep on it." This should be our response for any major decision whether it's business or personal.

Quite often business responsibilities for both men and women require a great deal of travel, and we all know that is no longer a joy ride. Travel entails long hours, inevitable lines everywhere, tight time schedules, less than perfect food, and not always the most comfortable bed.

Now we have an extra burden, and a heavy one at that. We have to be concerned about terrorist's attacks in America, and if you travel overseas, simply being an American presents a concern. This is something we never dreamed we would ever have to experience.

In an effort to handle all the responsibilities and challenges that business presents us, sleep deprivation is almost a given. Soon we find that our sleep debt resembles the national debt, and getting it paid off appears to be just a sweet dream.

However, in time you are going to find that you have created a nightmare for yourself.

You may have financial debts that you are struggling to pay, and I can understand this. However, if you reduce your sleep debt first, you will find that you can handle all other debts in your life with less anxiety and a greatly improved attitude toward them.

According to the National Sleep Foundation's recent survey, *45% of the population admitted they are willing to sleep less in order to get more done.* This misguided 45% need to reverse their thinking, and realize they *could get more done if they slept more.*

You may think you're cheating sleep, but in reality, you're cheating yourself. If you're sleep deprived, you cannot live up to your potential in any area of your life.

Memory and focus are greatly reduced by sleep deprivation. Not only do we experience diminished mental acuity, but productivity, and quality of performance follow closely behind. Soon you have become a card-carrying member of the R&R Society. (Rush & Redo).

Many employers are now realizing the value of having well-rested and alert employees. In order to facilitate this new realization, they are providing "nap" areas for employees to take a ten-minute nap instead of a coffee break. What a brilliant decision!

I find this interesting because many years ago when I was an executive secretary in Chicago, this perk was available for the office staff, who wanted to take advantage of it. There was a small sofa in the coffee room. If you wanted to nap, you took your break at a time when the coffee room was not in use.

I don't mean to indicate that you should plan to catch up on your sleep at the office. Overcoming sleep deprivation is a personal responsibility that each of us has to handle. It becomes a matter of rearranging your priorities, and making a commitment.

The High Price of Sleep Deprivation

Sleep deprivation also creates an incredible number of accidents, not only on the highways, but in the workplace, as well. I alluded to some of the most publicized accidents earlier, and would like to reiterate them in the following quotation Rubin Naiman, Ph., Clinical Health Psychologist:

"A lot of men wear sleep deprivation as a badge of courage. Dozens of CEO's pride themselves on sleeping just four to five hours a night. What happens, though, is that your judgment disappears, and your perception is impaired.

Three-Mile Island, Chernobyl and the Exxon Valdez are all examples of sleep related accidents.

To remain healthy and at your peak, you need about eight hours of sleep per night. Einstein slept ten hours."

Don't allow yourself to become an accident waiting to happen, because of sleep deprivation. Remember that the Universe has a perfect accounting system, and all debts must be paid. If you neglect your health, you will pay with disease. If you neglect your sleep, you may pay with a stupid and costly mistake in your business. Even worse, you may pay with an accident on a highway that is fatal to you, someone you love, or someone you don't even know.

Please don't gamble with sleep deprivation. The odds are against you. The price is too high.

Defining Success

Much of society only defines success in terms of financial achievement. Certainly, we kid ourselves if we think money doesn't matter. It does. However, we also have to put money in the proper perspective. It isn't very satisfying to have to spend the money you worked so hard to earn on health care, which is currently off the Richter scale. Remember that sleep deprivation not only diminishes the quality of your life by putting you at risk for heart attacks, a weakened immune system, obesity and diabetes, but it also shortens your life.

What joy can you find in financial success if you've ruined your health and destroyed valuable relationships along the way? Believe me, I'm not trying to take anyone on a guilt trip. I know that most people want more for their loved ones, and quite often this is the driving force behind all the long hours. I'm only attempting to enlighten you on the value of taking a serious look at your lifestyle, which is the reason for sleep deprivation about 50% of the time.

Making it all happen!

Very few people love the "sweet smell of success" more than I do. However, one thing I have learned is that it has to be approached from an entirely different perspective than I used to, and than most people do. Quite often success is elusive, *not because it is not possible*, but because we have tried to work harder, instead of smarter.

The world is full of wonderful human beings who have worked long hours at a job or in a business, year after year. They have denied themselves time with their family and friends, only to discover in the end that they have very little to show for their efforts.

The most valuable lesson you must learn about success, is that it only happens <u>when you have your mind under control.</u> Your thoughts and feelings about yourself create your attitude. Your attitude controls your actions. When you have these all together, you have learned how to ADD.

Attitude+Direction+Discipline = SUCCESS!

You cannot have control over your thoughts, feelings and actions *without sufficient sleep.* I tried it for years. I can assure you, *it just doesn't work!*

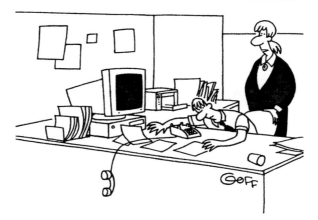

"It really impresses the customers
if you're awake when they call."

Finding Time to Sleep

*"But I have promises to keep,
and miles to go before I sleep."*

Robert Frost
American Poet
1874 – 1963

You may not have expected to find a time management chapter in a book on sleep. However, I have talked with so many people who tell me they could sleep, if they could only find the time to do so, that it seemed like an essential subject to address. Sleep deprivation doles out pretty much the same consequences, whether it is caused by pain, anxiety or lack of time.

There is just so much that has to be done each day. This is especially true of working mothers, even if modern dads pitch in and help more than has been the case in the past. If you're a single, working mother, it's even a bigger challenge. I know women in their thirties and forties who are trying to work full time jobs, further their education in order to get higher paying jobs, and are racked with guilt because they cannot spend as much time with their children as they want and feel they need to do. It's a terrible situation to be in, and sleep deprivation is almost a given.

Another area of great concern is the mother who is up numerous times in the night with a newborn, and yet has to be awake and alert during the day to care for older children, as well as the baby.

Recently, I was talking with my friend, Mickey Schlatter, who told me when her children were small, she told Bob, her husband, the nicest gift he could give her would be 24 hours in a motel, just so she could sleep without inter-ruptions. I would guess that there are quite a few young mothers out there who can relate to this. This might be something husbands would like to consider doing as a special gift. It doesn't have to be a five-star hotel, just a quiet place.

If you happen to be a stay-at-home mother, you might want to consider trading sleep time with someone you know well, who is in your same situation. Instead of trading baby-sitting time just for shopping, errands or social activities, give some thought to trading for a few hours of uninterrupted sleep. Even if you can only do this once a week, it would be of some help.

If it seems like I'm overly concerned about women finding the time to sleep, I am. Statistics show that they are the most sleep deprived. I don't mean to indicate that many men are not, because they are. It's just that most men can sleep anywhere, anytime, and women cannot do this. Men can sleep in front of a television, right through a war. You don't see a woman doing this. I see men sleeping in the car, or in a chair in a department store, while they are waiting for a woman who is shopping. All these little naps help a great deal to prevent sleep deprivation.

Caregivers are another concern. When they are tending to loved ones quite often they lose a lot of sleep at night. Yet they have to function competently during the day to continue with the care.

Then there are men and women who work long hours at a job, endure a frustrating commute, arrive home exhausted only to be faced with other family responsibilities, domestic duties, phone calls to return, bills to pay, and so forth. It seems endless.

As Brian Tracy tells us in his Time Management course, we are a time poverty nation. He says it's more prevalent than wealth poverty, because even the wealthy do not have enough time. In my opinion, this situation is created, to some degree, due to poor management, and I think a lot of people who are not considered to be "wealthy" would concur. If you have ample money, you can certainly hire a considerable amount of help to handle the non-essential tasks. This is a privilege not everyone has at their disposal.

Unfortunately, a lot of time is wasted. Now there may be some resistance to this statement but it's a fact of life. Benjamin Franklin said, "Do you love life? Then don't squander time, because that's the stuff life is made of." This is so true, yet most of us do not really take this into consideration. Your time is very valuable, and you should consider it so. When you waste your time, it's just like wasting your money. Neither of these habits is intelligent nor admirable.

Most of us do not realize that we have been wasting time, because we are so engrained with the habits of society, and our acceptance of this type of lifestyle. I must point out though, if you truly want to change the results in your life, so that you can get more sleep, have more energy and are healthier, happier, and more productive, (and therefore more successful) it's imperative that you begin making some changes in your lifestyle. A time management program will indisputably change your life for the better. In fact, Brian Tracy points out in his Time Management seminar that "The quality of your life is largely determined by the quality of your time management."

Becoming a good time manager is an entire course in itself, and I highly recommend that you look into it, even though you may think you do not have time to take on any other projects. I can almost guarantee you that a good time management course would point out at least a few areas where you could help yourself find more time. A wise man once said, "The best explanation of insanity is doing the same thing over and over again, and expecting a different result." Therefore, if your life isn't working out the way you want it to, and you truly want better results, like finding more time to sleep, you absolutely have to look into ways that you can do things differently. You cannot continue on the same path you've been on, and expect to arrive at a different destination. It just can't be done.

Buy, or borrow from your local library, a good time management course. I have mentioned Brian Tracy's Time Management because this is the one I used, and found it very helpful. Get a Sony Walkman or regular tape player and listen to the tapes while you work around the house, in your car, walking or other activities. One of the fastest ways to find more time is to **listen rather than watch.** Television consumes an enormous amount of time. Even if you think you're just listening, chances are pretty good that you'll find yourself "taking a peek" at the screen, and end up watching for five minutes or more. This action also distracts your focus, which listening does not do.

The first step you need to take in order to find more time to sleep is to make sleep a priority. We always find time for our priorities. Do I hear you saying, but sleep isn't a priority? Well, you might want to rethink your priorities, as well as go over some of the downside issues of sleep deprivation. In fact, let me list a few right now, so you don't have to take the time to go back and search them out:

Over 100,000 accidents, 71,000 injuries, 1,550 deaths occur each year in the United States alone due to drowsy drivers (National Sleep Foundation's survey).

A weakened immune system. Our immune system works very hard while we're asleep. Did you ever consider that this is why you feel better the next morning? I'm sure everyone has experienced this whether it's recovering from a cold, the flu or other illnesses. I've talked with patients recovering from cancer who have been adamant about the critical role ample sleep has played in the healing process.

Increased risk for heart attacks, obesity, diabetes and other related diseases.

Premature aging, wrinkled skin, poor muscle tone, poor posture, lack of vitality and zest for life.

Depression, lack of the ability to handle stress, poor memory, low energy, short tempers, road rage, poor work performance and productivity have all been associated with sleep deprivation.

Do you need more?

Decreased libido and sexual performance. This should get your attention.

After you make sleep a priority, then you must make a commitment to take steps to rearrange your lifestyle in a manner that will be conducive to getting more sleep. Something magical happens when you make a commitment. All sorts of wonderful things come into your life to help you to manifest the commitment. Don't ask me how, I just know that it happens.

Following priority and commitment come actions. Here are a few areas you might want to consider when creating your new lifestyle and finding ways to get more sleep.

Have a family board meeting.

Sit down with your entire family and go over the advantages of sleep for not only yourself and other adults, but for children and teens, as well. It may be harder to sell teens on the idea of better productivity, but most of them are interested in their appearance. Certainly ample sleep creates a more beautiful complexion and sparkling eyes. That's why we call it beauty sleep. It also greatly enhances sports performance, which should be of interest to your sports jock. Any serious athlete knows the value of sufficient sleep.

Also discuss the downside of sleep deprivation with them, the accidents, poor memory for school tests, etc.

You might want to explain the benefits of a more pleasant environment in school, the office and especially at home. People are happier, more patient, more caring and listen to others more intently when they are not tired.

Get everyone involved to make this new lifestyle a joy rather than a challenge, and that is exactly what it will be, a JOY. When people are involved in a project, they take an interest in its success. Once everyone starts enjoying the benefits, the momentum grows.

Make household duties a family affair. After all, the entire family lives there.

This is sometimes a challenge because not everyone wants to have things as neat as others in the family. It might be a good idea to try to drop, or at least tone-down perfectionism, and learn to live with a less than perfect house. However, keep in mind that clutter creates chaos. If each family member learns to pick up his own clothes, put things away after using them, and pitch in with just one or two small weekly duties, it will be amazing how organized a house can be with very little effort. It isn't necessary to have every speck of dust removed, but it is time consuming and frustrating when items are buried in clutter, and difficult to find. More time goes into hunting for lost items than anyone would imagine.

Creative procrastination is quite different from general procrastination.

Creative procrastination works well with a lot of household duties. This is a term I learned from Brian Tracy, and have been trying to implement into my life. I prefer to have things clean, neat and in order at all times. So much for toning down perfectionism. However, I have finally learned (the hard way) that there is never enough time to do everything. Therefore, I have started to ask myself, "Is this moving me toward my goal?" "Does this have to be done now?" "What are the disadvantages of doing it next week, rather than today?" The benefits that come from creative procrastination is that a lot of things you thought had to be done, just went away in a week, or at least did not get any worse by waiting for a week. This might entail household duties like sweeping the patio or raking the yard. You may not like the way the yard looks with leaves, but chances are pretty good that it won't hurt anything, and you have gained an hour or so by doing it every other week rather than every week. Get the idea? Keep in mind though, it's crucial for you to use that extra time to do something constructive that will help you get to bed earlier.

Budget your time for different projects.

Good time managers look at time in increments of minutes, rather than hours. Also when you budget your time, you have a tendency to work with more urgency than otherwise. It's important to develop a sense of urgency about life in general. People who make things move in this world share the same sense of urgency. Believe me, I am not trying to program you for more stress by suggesting that you develop a sense of urgency. It's just that you accomplish more when you move faster, and your mind is more focused on what you're doing than if you're just moping along in a hapless fashion. The more you accomplish in a short period of time, the more time you have to do the things that make life enjoyable. Plus, accomplishment creates energy, and enthusiasm.

Please keep in mind as you develop a sense of urgency, this does not mean you do not take time to relax, reflect and meditate. It's very important that you do this. Otherwise, your mind will become exhausted.

Organize and simplify.

Take time on the weekend to organize the following week. This goes for anything that has to be done from menu planning, grocery shopping and errands to organizing clothes for work and school, as well as household duties. It may be difficult to find the time to do this at first.

However, once you do it, you'll be so amazed at how smooth the following week runs, that it will become a priority.

If you create a revolving set of menus for a month or six weeks, you will find it easier to come up with meal ideas, and you will be more organized in your food shopping, because you know what you need for each meal. This does not mean you cannot deviate from time to time, but it certainly helps to know a week in advance what you will serve for dinner each night. It can get very stressful if you have to come up with different and interesting meal ideas every day, after you get home from work. Quite often people end up eating whatever is easiest, and fastest, rather than what is best for health and vitality. Also if you have the weekly menu announced and posted, it eliminates your spouse having pasta for lunch on the same day you were planning it for dinner.

If you know what you and your children will wear each day of the week, it will save last minute emergency washing and ironing, as well as a crisis in the morning when everyone is trying to rush out of the house.

Make a list.

Working from a daily list will save you more time than you can imagine. I was very rebellious about this in the beginning. I used to insist, "I don't have time to write things down. Every minute is filled, and I run from one project to the other. I don't need a list. I already know what has to be done."

Well, I must tell you, I was wrong. Once you learn to work from a list, you will be amazed at how much more you will accomplish. Even more importantly, you will be doing the things that really need to be done, rather than the thousands of urgent things that are always screaming to be done.

Certainly there will be times when you must tend to urgent things, and sometimes a project may be both urgent and important. This, of course, is the best place to spend your time. However, more often than not, we tend to do things that seem urgent, but are really not very important in the scheme of things.

Bob Proctor is one of my most valued mentors. I have learned so much from him about understanding how the mind works, making money and setting goals. One thing he shared with us in his Goal Achiever Seminar program is that we should list only **six** items that need to be done the next day, put them in order of their importance, and don't do anything else until those six items are completed.

I used to list 12 or 16 items, get confused

about what should be done first, and frustrated by the end of the day, because so many things did not get done. Keep in mind, if you have one project that will take three to five hours, then don't make yourself crazy by listing six projects. But make sure the projects you list are "goal-oriented" projects ... activities that will move you closer to your goal and not just a "To Do" list.

However, this "six list" is an invaluable time saver and productivity tool. In his Goal Achiever Seminar, Bob shared with us that Charles Schwab paid $25,000 for this idea. His office was not accomplishing what they knew they needed to do. They did not need new ways to do things, but rather a method of getting done what they already knew they should do. The "six list" worked for them and has worked for thousands of people since. I think you too will find this a very helpful time management tool.

By the way, I highly recommend that you look into Bob Proctor's "The Goal Achiever" program. He gives you complete details on how to use the "six list" and a myriad of other ideas. If you follow the advice he gives you, your life will change in ways you cannot imagine. See the Resource Directory.

Learn to say NO.

I know women who are stretched to the max with their time, because they say "yes," to every request that comes up. Once people realize you're a "yes" person, you will be asked to serve on every board, help out with every school or church project, and fundraiser. Every family member who wants help will come to you, as well as every friend in your address book. Although saying yes may seem admirable, and should be done at times, it isn't fair to yourself, or your loved ones, to be spread so thin. In fact, it may even be a sign of low self-esteem, which is never healthy.

If you're a "yes" person, you might consider that you can say "no" to the project, and yet say "yes" to the person asking for your help. Perhaps you can make a donation of money, rather than your time, or say that you cannot do it now, but ask them to keep you in mind later, and to give you some advance notice so you can schedule it.

Most people truly do understand. Especially if you explain in a kind and caring fashion.

Quick Tips

Every home should have a file cabinet whether it's the base for a business or not. File cabinets can save a great amount of time for daily activities. One tip that has helped me a great deal is to get different colored hanging files. Write on the tab indexes (that go in the plastic slots) Sunday, Monday, Tuesday, etc. You should have one for every day of the week. Separate the tabs so that each day is clearly visible.

Next make up files for the twelve months of the year. Use these files to put in anything that needs to be done on certain days, and in certain months. They are great to use for storage of letters, articles or projects that cannot be handled on the spot. If I know I can't get to something on Monday, and it won't create a problem to postpone it, I may drop it in Wednesday or Friday. This way it's off my desk, and out of my mind. I don't have to worry about remembering it, because I'll see it when I open Friday's file.

Do the same with items you may not want to make a decision on until several months down the road. Put it in the file of the month when you want to consider it, and forget it. It's very freeing.

Until you get into the habit of pulling out your monthly files the first of each month, you may want to put a post note on your calendar that reminds you to do this. Just write, "Pull monthly file." You can use the same note from month to month simply by transferring it on to the following calendar page.

Check your telephone time.

How much time are you spending on the telephone in friendly but somewhat idle chatter? Please don't misunderstand me. Keeping in touch with family and true friends is an extremely important part of life. However, I don't recommend spending a lot of time with the woman who used to live next door, who you didn't really care all that much about, but has called to tell you about her gall bladder operation.

I'm not suggesting that you be rude, but remember, there are only 24 hours in a day. Are you better off to cut her time down considerably, and get an additional 15 minutes of sleep? It's something to think about.

Get off the phone with telemarketers immediately. I quickly tell them that I know they have a very difficult job, (which they do) and I don't want to take their time to explain anything to me, because I'm not interested. Hang up.

Monitor Television time.

This is a real time consumer. There are hundreds of valuable educational programs on television. There are just as many extremely entertaining and life enhancing shows available for us to watch and enjoy, and I suggest that you schedule some of these into your lifestyle.

Much of our population spends countless hours in front of the television watching mindless shows that they don't even remember the next morning, many of which have toxic scripts and performances. It is just so pointless to spend your precious time in this manner. If you really need to escape from your current world, watch something that is inspiring and uplifting, that will motivate you to take steps to get yourself out of your current situation.

However, be sure to be an action person. Don't spend so much time getting motivated that there is no time for action.

We all think we're too busy to get more sleep. This has been a major reason people have given me for their sleep deprivation. Yet research surveys indicate that in many homes in American, television is watched **40 hours per week.** Just think what could be accomplished, and how lives could be changed for the better if even half of this time would be used for additional sleep, and other constructive projects.

Making downtime work for you.

Always carry a note pad and pen with you. I like a spiral pad with a heavy cover so it's easy to write anywhere. You can work on duty lists, shopping lists, or daydream with your goal list. Every time you write down your goals, they become stronger in your subconscious mind, which moves you closer to ideas of accomplishment.

Use your cell phone to return quick phone calls and to make appointments for the dentist, or hairdresser, etc. Make sure you have a calendar or appointment book with you so you can jot down the time and date. It's so nice to have these little tasks out of the way when you get home.

If you walk, cell phones are very handy to get some of your other calls made. I don't like to use my entire walk time on a cell phone, as it's extremely important to me to use this time to communicate with nature, and it should be to you as well. If you have a beautiful park to walk in, as I do, it's a crime to ignore the environment. However, if time allows for both, this is a more productive way to talk to family and friends than just sitting at a desk. At least you're getting some exercise.

Create a downtime reading file. Put magazine, newspaper articles or mail that you have not had time to read in this file. Read these items when you're standing in line at the post office or bank, rather than mindlessly paging through a two year old magazine in the doctor's office.

I'm sure, if you give it some thought, you can come up with time saving ideas that fit into your personal lifestyle. Make it a game, and make it fun. See who in the family can come up with the most and best ideas for saving time. Give a special prize to the one who does it. This will get everyone involved, and everyone will benefit from having more time to sleep.

Many people give far more attention to arranging time in their lives for a vacation or other social activities, than they do to getting enough sleep. Yet, with sufficient sleep, every day is more relaxed and enjoyable. However, without enough sleep, even the most exciting and expensive vacation lacks luster.

Please know that I am fully aware of the

challenges of finding time to get sufficient sleep. I was sleep deprived for many years, not only from lack of time, working 60-70 hours a week in a struggling business, but from the anxiety that went with the territory. Perhaps this is why I'm so adamant about trying to help others look at their priorities in a different light. I can guarantee you, if I had it to do over, it would not be handled the same way. I was just so accustomed to being sleep deprived that I accepted it as a way of life. I don't want you to make the same mistake.

CHAPTER 11

♋♋

Rest
For The
Weary

ﺏﺏ

*"It seemed to be a necessary ritual that
he should prepare himself for sleep, by
meditating under the solemnity of the
night sky . . . a mysterious transition
between the infinity of the soul and
the infinity of the universe."*

Victor Hugo
French Poet / Novelist
1802 – 1885

Creating a bedtime ritual is an important step
to regular and restful sleep. Too often, with our
busy schedules we think we can work until the
minute we drop into bed. This routine is not
conducive to anything satisfactory in the bedroom.
You can't just jump in the bed and enjoy peaceful

sleep, any more than you can just jump in bed and experience sex to its greatest potential. If a successful outcome is the goal, then you have to understand that both of these activities depend on a relaxed mind.

Each person must try to develop a bedtime ritual that can be maintained, at least, the majority of the time. Certainly, there will be times in our lives when we have circumstances that absolutely deny us this gift to ourselves, and will probably also deny us sleep. However, if a quieting down routine is established, as a habit, it will undoubtedly amaze you how you manage to get it worked into a busy schedule.

The purpose of this quieting down routine is to establish a chain of activities that prepare you for sleep.

I would like to suggest that you begin by turning down the noise in your home. Turn off the television, radio and other noise polluters. Beautiful calm music greatly enhances a bedtime ritual.

Not everyone is comfortable with turning off the phone. However, if you have an answering machine, and an emergency number you can leave with family, it is relaxing to know that the phone isn't going to interrupt your meditation or quiet hour. It's amazing how "out of the blue" someone that you haven't heard from in months or maybe years, will decide to give you a call on a Tuesday night around 9:30.

Turn down the lights in the bedroom, and in the bathroom. It's emotionally soothing to take a bath by candlelight. If you're careless about candles then use a small nightlight. You get the same effect.

When you're in your bath (or shower), be kind to yourself. Bathe your body with love and appreciation. It is, after all, a creation of the Divine Creator. If you have abused and neglected it, then this is a good time for you to start rectifying these mistakes.

Also, while you're in your bath, be judicious about your thoughts. Think about wonderful things in your life. This would be a great time to recite your gratitude list, or think about someone you love, and how blessed you are to have him or her in your life.

Don't allow the activities of the day to intrude on this quiet sanctuary you have carved out for yourself. Remember, ONLY YOU can accept, or reject thoughts that go into your mind. I read in "O" Magazine, "What you find in your mind, is what *you* put there. Put good things there." That's gospel truth, if I've ever heard it.

After your bath routine, you might want to do some slow, relaxing stretches, yoga or tai chi movements to increase flexibility. Your muscles will be relaxed and willing to stretch.

Wear the most comfortable, sensuous clothes to bed possible. Even better, wear nothing to bed. Sleeping in the nude not only makes you feel totally free, but it is wonderful for your skin, as it gets an "air bath." Plus, you never get twisted up in nightclothes.

Now is a nice time to have a cup of Bedtime tea, or Chamomile, both of which are calming. While you have your tea, read something inspirational, spiritual and reassuring. If you did not recite your gratitude list in the tub, do it now. It's important to do this often.

I cannot be too emphatic about the importance of thanking God for your gifts. We acknowledge our blessings too little, and complain too much. We need to get this habit turned around.

After tea, comes meditation and prayer, and after that . . . turn out the lights and enjoy soothing, restful slumber! Sweet Dreams.

I'm sure that this bedtime ritual is not going to work for everyone. I know when you have children to bathe and get to bed, a load of laundry to do after that, and heaven only knows what else, that the above routine seems like I think you live in a fantasy world. I don't! I just want to give you some suggestions that hopefully you can implement some of the time. Maybe you have to start with only a few ideas, but do start. You might want to ask yourself... if not now, when? The life you're living is not a dress rehearsal... this is the real thing!

You have to *make* quiet time for yourself. I can guarantee you no one else will do it for you. *You deserve it.*

CHAPTER 12

Snoring

*"Laugh and the world laughs with you.
Snore and you sleep alone."*

Anthony Burgess
British Novelist/London Critic
1917 – 1993

A snoring partner can create more consistent and continuous sleep deprivation than perhaps any other cause. This is a very delicate subject, because it is sometimes difficult to come to grips with. We have to deal with denial (I don't snore), egos, excuses, and perhaps unidentified more serious sleep disorders.

Most people who snore are overweight, middle-aged, and male. This difference is adjusted after menopause. However, compared to women, men snore more, and are eight times as likely to develop sleep apnea, which is a serious sleep disorder. This may sound alarming, but according to Dr. James Maas, only 1 out of 100 snorers suffer from sleep apnea, yet between 30-40% of adults snore. If snoring seems to be very loud, and there is an abnormal breathing pattern, you should check with a physician.

Research indicates that you may be more inclined to snore if other people in your family were snorers. Many people snore occasionally. It's the chronic snorers that create havoc.

Usually snoring is not a serious problem, and can be eliminated or at least greatly improved by following some or all of the suggestions below.

Lose weight.

Shedding excess fat has been shown to substantially decrease, if not eliminate, snoring. Even being 10 pounds overweight, can create a snoring problem.

Better sleep posture.

Sleeping on one's back can cause snoring. Sleep experts recommend using a cervical support pillow, which has been found to reduce snoring. This keeps your head up, and the airways open. It is also helpful to sleep on one's side. See Appendix for pillow information.

Avoid sleeping pills and sedatives.

They put you to sleep, but when you're very relaxed, the muscles also slacken, and make snoring worse.

Avoid late snacks and alcoholic beverages.
Both contribute to snoring, as they relax the muscles.

Dr. Edzard Ernst, M.D. recommends singing. He says singing or humming firms up flabby muscles in the upper airways. If you can't sing, hum a few bars, twenty minutes per day.

Herbal decongestants have been used for many years for sleep aids. A couple that seem to help with snoring are bromelain (an enzyme extracted from pineapple), and citrus aurantium (bitter orange) derived from the Chinese fruit, zhishi.

Natural lubricants such as almond oil, olive oil or eucalyptus oil can be sprayed toward the back of the tongue. While these are more anecdotal than scientific, it's worth a try.

Take the time to sit down and discuss this problem with your partner, so you can work out a solution. Sometimes separate bedrooms are necessary to assure the non-snoring partner a good night's sleep. It is not fair, nor wise for the non-snoring partner to go through life sleep deprived, ruining their health and accelerating aging. Your snoring partner will be healthier too, if the snoring stops.

CHAPTER 13

〜✿〜

Sleep Disorders

〜✿〜

"Oh sleep! O gentle sleep!
Nature's soft nurse, how have I frighted thee,
That thou no more wilt weigh mine eyelids down
And steep my senses in forgetfulness? "

Henry Wadsworth Longfellow
U.S. Poet
1807 – 1882

Depending on how scientifically detailed you want to be, there are many different types of sleep disorders...well over fifty. However, we are going to list and discuss very briefly the most common.

INSOMNIA

There are many types of *insomnia*, and a variety of solutions. We have discussed general insomnia and solutions in earlier chapters. Basically, if you aren't sleeping for whatever cause, you're experiencing insomnia syndrome.

Don't allow insomnia to become a habit. After a few sleepless nights, some people begin to panic, and feel like they may never get a good night's sleep in the future. This can be self-fulfilling, and sleep problems begin to take on a life of their own. Don't ignore the situation, as it will only get worse. Take steps to correct it immediately, not three years down the road.

"Nothing cures insomnia like the realization that it's time to get up." *Unknown*

SLEEP APNEA

This is a serious sleep disorder. Symptoms are loud snoring, frequent episodes of stopped breathing, and then a gasp for breath. This pattern can repeat itself hundreds of times during the night, which thoroughly disrupts the normal sleep cycles.

This condition puts a dramatic strain on the heart, increasing the risk of heart attacks or strokes.

Individuals suffering from sleep apnea are frequently older, overweight men but it does affect women, as well. High blood pressure is also associated with sleep apnea.

NARCOLEPSY

Narcolepsy is somewhat unusual compared with *sleep apnea,* and is very serious. It is believed to be caused by a brain abnormality that is most likely inherited.

This sleep disorder involves excessive daytime sleepiness and "sleep attacks", which produce temporary muscle paralysis (such as in REM sleep).

The individual can actually collapse on the floor, and not be able to move for several minutes. These attacks can occur at anytime, but sometimes are brought on by strong emotions.

As you can see, this is a very debilitating disorder, and can be extremely dangerous. It needs to be diagnosed in a sleep center and treated with medication.

RESTLESS LEG SNYDROME

This sleep disorder is characterized by creeping, crawling, tingling or pain in the lower legs. These unpleasant and uncomfortable physical reactions occur as soon as the person tries to get to sleep. Symptoms can usually be relieved by stretching, or getting up and moving around. Also massage or a shower may help. Unfortunately, if you have to go through all of this, you're probably wide awake by the time you're finished with the chosen solution.

A related syndrome is *Periodic Leg Movement.* This is characterized by twitching and jerking during the night, which is severe enough to wake both the sufferer and the sleep partner.

There is a list of helpful web sites in the Resource Directory. Some of these will cover sleep research centers in general and others will be centers that specialize in specific sleep disorders.

CHAPTER 14

Your
Personal
Sleep Log

You might want to use the following page as a guideline to create a personal sleep diary. This is just a suggested format to give you some idea of what you should be considering when you create it.

Date _____

The time you went to bed _____

Did you fall asleep immediately? _____

How long do you think it took to get to sleep?
_____

How many times were you awake during the night?
_____

Did you go back to sleep promptly? _____

If not, how long were you awake? _____

What time did you get up? _____

Did you feel rested or tired in the morning?
_____

Did this fatigue leave later in the day? _____

Make a note of your evening routine, whether you slept well or poorly. This will enable you to either follow or eliminate some of the factors that may have had an impact on the quality and quantity of your sleep.

Sometimes factors that effect our sleep are temporary and do not indicate there is a major sleep problem, but will definitely change your sleep patterns. This can involve difficult decisions, grief, temporary pain, illness, a tight work schedule, or just being very excited about what is going on in your life.

Try to ride out this time the best you can. Use the sleep aids suggested in the chapter Healthy Natural Sleep Aids. Get in as many naps as life will allow, and don't work yourself into a frenzy. This will only make matters worse.

THESE ARE SOME OF THE QUESTIONS YOU SHOULD CONSIDER IF YOU DID NOT SLEEP WELL.

Did you take time to wind down and relax before bed?

Did you meditate and pray?

Did you exercise late in the day?

What did you eat before bed?

How much caffeine did you consume during the day?

What time did you have the last caffeine?

Were you on the telephone? Was the conversation upsetting?

Did you watch television before bed?

Were you on the computer until it was time to fall into bed?

Did you work late into the evening? Pay bills?

Was your day unusually stressful?

Are you trying to make major decisions in your life?

Did you have an upsetting conversation with someone you love, or maybe just a close friend?

Was the bedroom too hot, too light, too noisy?

Notes

_____

_____

_____

_____

_____

_____

_____

Notes

_____

_____

_____

_____

_____

_____

_____

CONCLUSION

Before you turn out the lights.....

Thank you for investing your time
and money in this book.

It is my sincere hope it has provided
you with some solutions to your sleep
deprivation problems, and that you feel
your investment has been a wise and
rewarding one.

I welcome your comments,
suggestions and sleep stories. Please
write me at the address found in the
Resource Directory under Author
Contact, or at Ronnoco Publishing.

Sweet Dreams!

119

RESOURCE DIRECTORY

Author Contact
fawn@fawnoconnor.com
www.facesaverpillow.com

Cartoons
Ted Goff, cartoonist
www.tedgoff.com

Face-Saver Pillow
Ageless Achievement
PO Box 403
Placentia, CA 92871
www.facesaverpillow.com

Facial Muscles Sketch
Send a Self-addressed, <u>stamped #10 envelope</u>
Ageless Achievement
PO Box 403
Placentia, CA 92871

Healthy, Natural Seep Aids
You should be able to find most of the herbs, vitamins, minerals and protein supplements at your local health store. If they are not available, and the store does not want to special order for you, try the following, or contact the author for further assistance.

Amino Fuel
Twin Laboratories
1-800-645-5626

Bed Time Tea
Trader Joe's
1-800-746-7858

Calorad
Ageless Achievement
714-996-5097
info@agelessachievement.com

KavaTone
Enzymatic Therapy
1-800-783-2286

Natural Calm
Natural Vitality
1-800-446-7462
info@vites.com

Let's Live Magazine
310-445-7500
info@letslivemag.com

- *Mentors* - *Alphabetically listed*

Canfield, Jack
www.jackcanfield.com

Dyer, Wayne
www.waynedyer.com

Hansen, Mark Victor
www.markvictorhansen.com

Kersey, Cynthia
www.unstoppable.net

Poynter, Dan
www.parapublishing.com

Proctor, Bob
www.bobproctor.com

Robbins, Anthony
www.anthonyrobbins.com

Rohn, Jim
www.jimrohn.com

Tracy, Brian
www.briantracy.com

Walters, Dottie
www.Walters-Intl.com

Zigler, Zig
www.zigzigler.com

Neck Pillow/Cervical Support
Ageless Achievement
PO Box 403, Placentia, CA 92871
info@facesaverpillow.com
www.facesaverpillow.com

Oxygen, The Answer by Tonita de'Raye
Ageless Achievement
PO Box 403, Placentia, CA 92871
info@agelessachievement.com

Sleep Organizations

A.P.N.E.A. NET
www.apneanet.org

National Sleep Foundation
www.sleepfoundation.org

SleepNet
www.sleepnet.com

Subliminal Message Cassettes
Ageless Achievement
PO Box 403, Placentia, CA 92871
714-996-5097
info@agelessachievement.com

Recommended Reading
The Promise of Sleep – William C. Dement, M.D.
Power Sleep – Dr. James B. Maas
How To Sleep Soundly Tonight – Barbara L. Heller, M.S.W.
Deep Sleep – John R. Haravey, Ph.D.

ৎৡ

NATIONAL SLEEP FOUNDATION

The National Sleep Foundation is a nonprofit organization dedicated to improving public health and safety by achieving greater understanding of sleep and sleep disorders.

The results of their research and surveys are helpful to all of us, since we all need sleep. There is a plethora of information on their web site -- not only statistics, but links to sleep centers for help, etc. Visit http://www.sleepfoundation.org.

Also, you might want to consider becoming a member, which is as low as $25.00 per year, and includes a subscription to "sleepmatters", a quarterly publication. Call 202-347-3471, Fax 202-347-3472 or you can subscribe online.

Maybe if we all get involved, we can change the attitude about sleep in this nation . . . and wouldn't we all be better off if that would happened!

❧❧

Guidebook For Your Subliminal Message Cassettes

❧❧

GUIDEBOOK FOR YOUR SUBLIMINAL MESSAGE CASSETTES

"Subliminal" means below the level of conscious awareness. Subliminal messages are statements which you don't consciously perceive with your senses, but which are received by the unconscious, or what we like to refer to as the "super-conscious" portion of your mind. Hundreds of research studies prove that the subconscious/super-conscious mind absorbs stimuli, which are missed by the conscious mind. Subliminal tapes contain positive suggestions, which directly influence the very powerful subconscious mind to help you make positive changes in your life.

The effectiveness of subliminal tapes lies in the fact that they reach the subconscious mind, which is the seat of all memories, knowledge and emotions. The unconscious mind has a powerful influence on conscious actions, thoughts, feelings, habits and behaviors, and actually controls and guides your life. If you want to make real, lasting changes and improvements in any areas of your life, you must first reach the subconscious mind where the changes begin.

THIS IS NOT HYPNOSIS OR VISUALIZATION

Subliminal tapes do not make use of hypnosis, visualization or meditative techniques, but instead contain powerful "programming" phrases subliminally recorded behind music and/or environmental sounds. YOU WILL NOT CONSCIOUSLY HEAR ANY SPOKEN WORDS ON THE TAPES. However, carefully selected words, phrases and statements designed to obtain the specific results desired are presented clearly to the subconscious mind. Your subconscious mind perceives thousands of positive suggestions condensed into each hour of recording time.

HOW TO USE SUBLIMINAL TAPES

Simply play the tapes, and enjoy the music or environmental sounds! No concentration or active effort is required for subliminal programs to be effective. Enjoy the soothing sounds as often as you desire, as you go about your daily activities. Subliminal tapes are effectively played while you're working, driving, reading, exercising, watching TV, listening to the radio, relaxing, or as you fall asleep.

Note: It is not absolutely necessary to use headphones when listening to your subliminal tapes in order to make them effective. However, I think you may find you will experience results a little faster if you use them. One reason is that you don't have your tape playing in one room, and then walk into another room, and miss part of the message. If you're a person who seems to be in motion most of the time, as I am, it's helpful to carry the message with you. This is only a personal observation.

I do not use headphones in the evening while listening to my Sleep Like A Baby, or Peace of Mind tapes. I play them while I'm getting ready for bed, because I'm pretty much confined to my bathroom. They are very effective using them this way.

Also, *never use headphones while driving. It greatly impairs your ability to drive safely, and is against the law.*

GETTING RESULTS

A script is provided with each tape, so you know the exact recorded subliminal message. It is not necessary to read the script while listening to the tape, although to enhance effectiveness, we suggest you use statements on the scripts as positive affirmations, repeating them to yourself from time to time. Many clients have found it very helpful to read the script aloud once each day just before going to sleep at night.

To maximize results, research indicates that you must play your subliminal tape at least once a day. Personally, I like to play them much more frequently. Most of my tapes have a tropical ocean format, so I can play a tape over, and over, and over, never tiring of it. It actually becomes anonymous background that I don't even realize is there, except for the amazing results. The more often the tape is played, the faster and greater the effect. Because each person is unique and individual, results will vary from person to person. Sometimes results are experienced within the first few playings, while in other cases, it may take a few days. If the resistance is powerful, it can take several weeks to see change. However, be assured that if you faithfully use the tape on a regular, daily basis, RESULTS WILL COME.

Once you get started and see results, it will encourage you to make the time to carry this process even further. You will understand that thought control helps you to accomplish more in less time, and with less effort than without it. It's called working smarter, rather than harder.

PRODUCERS OF THESE TAPES

The company that provides us with these remarkable tapes is one of the most reliable and respected producers of this type of educational material. The tapes that we use were developed by

Jonathan Parker, Ph.D, and Eldon Taylor, Ph.D. Both men have extensive academic credentials, and are pioneers in the field of mind power and self-development.

JONATHAN PARKER

Jonathan Parker has a Bachelor's degree in Education, Chemistry, and Theology. A Master's Degree in Counseling, Psychology, and a Doctor of Philosophy in Human Behavior & Development. For over 30 years he has been a counselor, therapist, and is author of one of the largest self-development libraries in the world.

ELDON TAYLOR

Eldon Taylor's earliest work with subliminal information processing was performed at the Utah State Prison in 1986-87. The results were so remarkable among the group exposed to the tapes, they are now in standard use in Utah's prison system. He is regarded as one of the world's foremost authorities on subliminal information processing, and hold's doctorates in psychology and hypnotherapy.

OTHER SUBJECTS AVAILABLE

There are subliminal message tapes available for many subjects. However, we chose the following because we are addressing sleep problems. Sleep surveys indicate that anxiety is one of the most common causes for insomnia. People have anxiety over numerous areas of their lives. Finances, health, aging, and weight problems are some of the factors, responsible for destroying peace of mind and restful sleep.

WHAT YOUR SUBLIMINAL TAPE IS TELLING YOU

Listed below is a sampling of the positive affirmations recorded on the following subliminal tapes. The format we have chosen for Restful Slumber and Peace of Mind is Gentle Woodwinds. This is a sublime musical blend of flute, harp and woodwinds, enhanced by the serene nature sounds of gently flowing stream and birds. The format for the balance of these tapes is Tropical Ocean, which is quiet, peaceful and makes it comfortable to listen continuously, without the impression of repetition. Remember, the more frequently you hear the messages, the faster the results.

❖ **REFRESHING SLUMBER / SLEEP LIKE A BABY** – I can sleep deeply and naturally. I accept myself as a good sleeper. I naturally fall into a deep sleep. Yes, I do. I sleep a restful, natural sleep. I am happy. I am thankful for my restful sleep. My life flows with harmony. As I lie down to sleep, I feel safe, secure and calm. I expect good things in life. I relax and fall asleep quickly. I trust myself. I view my dreams as positive. Sleeping restores and revitalizes me, etc.

❖ **PEACE OF MIND** – I am peaceful and tranquil. My life is secure, and I am contented. Each day I become more of a relaxed and tranquil person. I have peace of mind and relaxed inner security.

I am in control of my life. I choose to be happy and peaceful. My life is harmonious and fulfilling. I dissolve all negativity in and around me. I am contented with life. There is more calmness, peace and tranquility in my life than ever before. There is peace and contentment within me. I feel composed, tranquil and at peace. Peace of mind is mine. I accept all good and pleasant experiences into my life. I radiate the inner strength of peace to all I meet. I attract peace, goodness and harmony. I am relaxed calm and at ease.

❖ **CREATING PROSPERITY AND ABUNDANCE** – I am prosperous. I am a child of the universe. I appreciate my success. I have many blessings. Abundance is naturally mine. I have many blessings. I focus on my blessings. I become a magnet attracting prosperity. I am already successful. I realize my prosperity.

Prosperity is attracted. My mind magnetically attracts prosperity. Prosperity is attracted to me. Abundance and prosperity flow to me now. I hold prosperous thoughts. I naturally receive. I visualize my prosperous reality. I deserve prosperity. I invest my time. I deserve money. I work hard. I deserve success. My energy is stored in money. I have more money. I am a magnet attracting prosperity. I use money in good ways. Money is good. I know abundance exists throughout nature. I give thanks for my blessings.

❖ **FOREVER YOUNG** – I am enough. I am strong. I am healthy. I am young. My body remembers, I remember. I remember youth. My body remembers youth. My cells are young and healthy. Life is a miracle. Life is wonderful. I am positive. I am enthusiastic. My hair grows fast. My hair grows thick. My abdominal muscles are strong. I stand erect. My skin is young. My mind is keen. Every day I improve.
I feel fantastic. I am confident. I feel great about myself. My cells rejuvenate me perfectly, etc.

❖ **OPTIMAL WEIGHT LOSS** – I am energetic. My body is conscious. My mind wills health. All excess fat is shed from me. I exercise. I visualize exercise. My body burns off fat. I respect myself. Food is not a reward. Food is not a tranquilizer. I image my ideal weight. Life is fun. I forgive myself. I forgive others. I am stress-free. I use food properly. My body creates perfection. Fat disappears. My metabolism is raised. Excess fat becomes heat and energy. I am physically healthy. I am emotionally healthy. I succeed, etc.

ARE YOU AGING YOUR FACE EVERY TIME YOU SLEEP??

FACE-SAVER PILLOW®
THE ORIGINAL "ANTI-AGING" PILLOW

"THE PERFECT PAMPER PILLOW FOR PERSONAL CARE"

- **Protects your face while you're sleeping**, so that you do not wake up with lines and wrinkles in your skin.

- **Protects your facial skin** from being pulled and stretched when you sleep on your side. Stretching is very damaging. As we mature, we have less elasticity in our skin, so it does not readily return to its original position.

- **Prevents muscle breakdown.** The average head weighs between seven and ten pounds, depending on gender and body type. Any amount of weight pressing on your face for hours at a time, on a regular basis creates muscle breakdown, and accelerates facial aging. Skin is attached to muscle, so as the muscles elongate, due to breakdown and the pull of gravity, the skin follows. This creates a tired and aging appearance. Using the FACE-SAVER PILLOW® will prevent this damage, which will eventually occur even with your taut faces.

- **Creates better head posture** by training you to sleep with your head pulled up from the cervical area. This gives you an immediate more youthful appearance, and helps prevent jowls.

- ADDITIONAL BENEFITS -

- **The FACE-SAVER PILLOW®** was originally designed to protect your face from aging. However, it has many other beneficial uses.

- **Improves oxygen intake** during sleep, because your face isn't buried in a pillow. Oxygen helps your cells renew, and eliminate toxins. Therefore, you will experience a higher level of energy in the morning.

- **Gives excellent cervical support** while sleeping on your back. It also supports your head, so that it will not tip to the side during sleep, which could create pressure on your face. Using the FACE-SAVER PILLOW® while reading, watching TV and traveling, will give you cervical support as well.

- **The perfect adjunct for patients of cosmetic surgery**, chemical peels, or laser treatments. It totally supports the weight of one's head, therefore protecting the face during the postoperative healing process. Equally important is the fact that it will protect your financial investment. If you're considering any type of professional procedure on your face, now is the time to train yourself to sleep on the FACE-SAVER PILLOW®.

- **Because of the size and ergonomic design**, it's very effective for proper leg and hip alignment while sleeping on your side. This is particularly important for people who may be overweight, or for pregnant women.

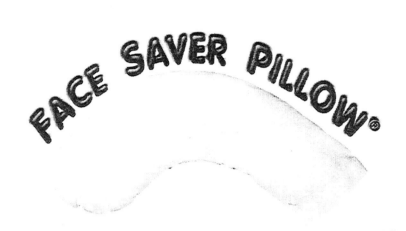

The FACE-SAVER PILLOW'S® ergonomic design provides not only great beauty benefits, but research indicates that it provides many health benefits, as well.

Since the average head weighs between seven to ten pounds, if you are sleeping on your face, you are sleeping lines and wrinkles into your skin. However, even more damaging is the breakdown of your muscle structure. Once this is broken down, gravity becomes very aggressive and elongates the muscles. Skin follows muscle, and you end up with a tired, aging appearance.

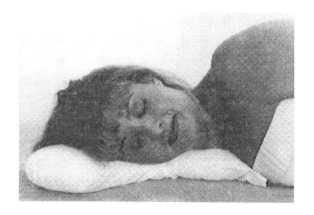

SLEEPING ON THE
FACE-SAVER PILLOW®

Prevents damage, because it bears the weight of your head, and allows your face to be suspended in air. When used properly, you should be able to slide your hand between your face and the mattress, or any sleeping surface, and not touch your face.

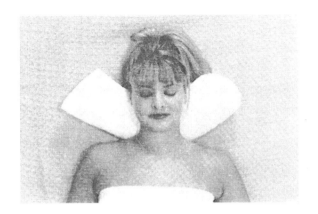

SUPREME
SUPPORT and COMFORT

Sleeping on your back with the FACE-SAVER PILLOW® not only gives you excellent cervical support, but it also supports your head. This prevents you from tilting your head to the side, which eliminates the tendency to sleep on the side of your face.